The Institute
Studies in B

The Physiology of Diving in Man and Other Animals

H. V. Hempleman
M.A., Ph.D.
Superintendent of the Royal Naval Physiological Laboratory

A. P. M. Lockwood
M.A., Ph.D., F.I.Biol.
Reader in Biological Oceanography,
The University of Southampton

Edward Arnold

Printed and bound in Great Britain at
The Camelot Press Ltd, Southampton

General Preface to the Series

It is no longer possible for one textbook to cover the whole field of Biology and to remain sufficiently up to date. At the same time teachers and students at school, college or university need to keep abreast of recent trends and know where the most significant developments are taking place.

To meet the need for this progressive approach the Institute of Biology has for some years sponsored this series of booklets dealing with subjects specially selected by a panel of editors. The enthusiastic acceptance of the series by teachers and students at school, college and university shows the usefulness of the books in providing a clear and up-to-date coverage of topics, particularly in areas of research and changing views.

Among features of the series are the attention given to methods, the inclusion of a selected list of books for further reading and, wherever possible, suggestions for practical work.

Readers' comments will be welcomed by the author or the Education Officer of the Institute.

1978

The Institute of Biology,
41 Queens Gate,
London, SW7 5HU

Preface

Man's envy of the specialist skills of other animals and his desire to explore the limits of the environment have proved powerful stimuli to technological progress and research.

The bottom of the deepest ocean trench has been reached by the Bathyscaphe but in respect to the duration of breath-holding dives or the simulated depths reached by divers unprotected from the external pressure by rigid containers, man was, until recently, hopelessly outclassed by the specialist diving mammals of the sea.

However, as more is learned of the physiological problems experienced by divers, many of the difficulties associated with prolonged deep diving have been overcome as is illustrated by the extension of safe open sea diving by man from a few minutes at 180 metres depth to many hours at 450 metres in the last ten years. Nevertheless, even the latter depth represents less than a quarter of that achieved by the sperm whale, doyen of the deep divers.

Our purpose here is to present an introduction to some of the capabilities of diving birds and mammals, to describe the physiological, biochemical and anatomical features which make prolonged submersion possible in air-breathing forms and to discuss the recent advances in man's diving techniques.

Portsmouth and Southampton, 1978

H. V. H.
A. P. M. L.

Contents

1 Introduction

One of the overriding fascinations of the marine mammals is their ability to remain submerged for extended periods of time and to dive to considerable depths.

Knowledge of the maximum diving capabilities of many species is still far from clear, but during the last fifty years it has become increasingly evident that the claims of the whalers of the last century, though scoffed at by the pundits of their day as exaggerated, were substantially correct.

At first, evidence for the depth achieved was based on the amount of line taken out by harpooned whales 'sounding' almost vertically, from a number of cases where individuals sustained injuries through striking the bottom and, in the case of diving birds, of specimens being caught in nets or crab pots set at known depths. More recently knowledge of the diving performance of seals and dolphins has been extended by use of sonar and depth-recording packs attached to the animals, though most of the available information naturally relates to the usual diving depths of the species studied rather than to their maximum capabilities.

Sperm whales, part of whose food often consists of animals living on or near the sea bed, are probably the deepest divers. Several have become entangled in cables at depths exceeding 800 m (2600 ft). The record depth at which this has occurred is 1134 m (3720 ft), more than ten times the maximum reported breath-holding dive achieved by man (100 m, 328 ft, Jacques Mayol, *Triton*, **22,** 148–9 and 201, 1977). However the sperm whale's limit may perhaps far exceed even 1100 m (3600 ft) since, if reliance may be placed on the depth distribution of squid species taken from whale stomachs, the cetacean may even reach 3000 m (9850 ft). Baleen whales rarely dive far but, when stressed, as by harpooning, they too may go to considerable depths (Table 1). The smaller cetaceans, dolphins and porpoises, do not generally dive deeply but a dolphin (*Tursiops truncatus*) trained to press a switch on a sonar beacon would voluntarily descend to 300 m (1000 ft) to locate the sound source. The Weddell seal, has been known to reach 600 m (1950 ft), thus rivalling some of the larger cetaceans. Among birds the emperor penguin sounds to 265 m (870 ft) but of the other scattered records, mostly based on birds caught in nets or crab pots, few are below 50 m (165 ft).

Of course, since marine mammals and birds are concerned with the primary task of locating their food rather than with establishing records, the great majority of dives are to lesser depths than those indicated above. Intensive study of the Weddell seal by G. L. Kooyman and his group has shown a distinct pattern of dives. This animal, which spends much of

Table 1   Maximum depths and dive times for selected diving mammals and birds.

	Depth (m)	Time (min)
Sperm whale (*Physeter catodon*)	1134	75
Bottlenose whale (*Hyperoodon rostratus*)	—	120
Finback whale (*Balaenoptera physalis*)	500	30
Blue whale (*Balaenoptera musculus*)	100	50
Dolphin (*Delphinus delphis*)	260	—
Bottlenose dolphin (*Tursiops truncatus*)	300	c. 15
Grey seal (*Halichoerus grypus*)	145	18
Weddell seal (*Leptonychotes weddelli*)	600	70
Beaver (*Castor canadensis*)	—	15
Emperor penguin (*Aptenodytes forsteri*)	265	18
Cormorant (*Phalacrocorax carbo*)	37	1.2
Penguin (*Pygoscelis*)	12	7

its life on or under the ice cover of Antarctic seas, apparently has two distinct purposes when submerged: (1) to find and capture food and (2) to locate new air holes through the ice where it can emerge to breathe. Separate forms of dive are associated with these activities: (a) fairly deep but relatively short excursions after prey and (b) dives which are longer both in duration and in distance travelled but which occur at relatively shallow depths below the ice (Fig. 1–1). Generally the deeper dives last about 6–15 min but much longer periods of submergence, up to 70 min, are associated with the search for air holes. The time which the Weddell

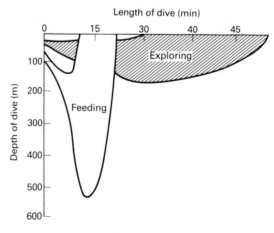

Fig. 1–1   Diving patterns of the Weddell seal. (After KOOYMAN, 1972.)

seal can withstand apnoea (absence of breathing) is long by the typical standards of seals, most of which can tolerate only about 20 min (Table 1), but even its performance is outdone by that of the bottlenose whale which has been reported to remain down for up to 120 min between successive 'blows' and by some reptiles which can submerge for days in shallow water. By comparison, man's ability to undertake active breath-holding dives is limited to some 2 or 4 min at most though R. Foster achieved a period underwater in an inactive state of 5 min 40 s. Mayol's 100 m dive lasted 3 min 39 s.

The difference in performance of the specialist diving forms and that of man and other terrestrial animals invites questions as to how diving species are adapted to enable them to remain below the surface so long and to tolerate the adverse effects likely to result from exposure to high hydrostatic pressure.

When any animal holds its breath or is denied access to air there is a decrease in oxygen and build up of CO_2 tension in its blood at rates determined by activity, body temperature, buffering capacity of the blood and size of the initial oxygen pool in the body. In man the higher centres of the brain can exert voluntary inhibition of the medullary respiratory centre when the CO_2 tension in the blood is low. As the CO_2 levels build up it becomes increasingly difficult for voluntary apnoea to be maintained and a diver is forced to the surface. Hypothetically therefore a specialist diving form might find it advantageous to increase the buffering capacity of its blood and to decrease the sensitivity of the respiratory centre to CO_2. Indeed both these factors do form part of the physiological repertoire of specialization of divers but they could not alone account for the prolongation of dives to the extent observed because of the effect of declining oxygen availability to sensitive tissues.

In terrestrial vertebrates the muscles and most of the visceral organs are comparatively tolerant of temporary O_2 lack but since the heart and brain are extremely sensitive, low oxygen tensions in the blood cannot be tolerated.

Several options would seem to be open in order to prolong the period of apnoea: (1) increase in the amount of oxygen carried down at the start of a dive: (2) decrease in metabolic rate to conserve oxygen during submergence; (3) decrease in the sensitivity of the central nervous system to oxygen lack; (4) circulatory re-routing of oxygenated blood to ensure that the more sensitive tissues receive sufficient oxygen; and (5) biochemical modification to improve energy production during anaerobic periods. To varying degrees all these modifications are utilized by diving species.

2 Oxygen Capacity of the Body

Oxygen is present in the body in three main areas: (a) in the lungs, sinuses and major airways, (b) in conjunction with the pigment haemoglobin in the blood and (c) in combination with the haemoglobin-like pigment, myoglobin, in the muscles.

2.1 Lung oxygen capacity

Seals have lungs with a volume comparable to that of man at about 5 litres per kg body weight. During a dive, however, seals probably derive less O_2 from the lung than does man since they tend to exhale prior to submerging. The oxygen availability from the lungs of deep-diving whales such as the bottlenose and fin is limited by two factors even though the animals dive after inhaling. Firstly, the lung volume, relative to body weight, is rather small by comparison with that of man. Secondly, the whale's lung appears to be structurally designed for ready collapse under the influence of raised hydrostatic pressure. Increasing pressure results in the compression of the flexible lungs and expulsion of the contained gas into the 'dead spaces' (i.e. non-respiratory regions) of the trachea and other main airways. These dead spaces (which tend to be structurally rather rigid) have a volume equivalent of some 10% of the lung volume at the surface. Consequently, assuming that Boyle's law operates, and that hydrostatic pressure increases at approximately one atmosphere for each 10 m (33 ft) depth* it would be expected that all or almost all, of the lung gas would have been forced into the airways by the time the animals reach a depth of c. 100 m (330 ft) (i.e. 11 atmospheres absolute (ATA)). Gas thus removed from contact with the respiratory surfaces in the alveoli will not be available for respiratory purposes in deeper parts of the dive.

However, when the animal approaches shallower depths during the concluding stages of a dive the gas will again enter the alveoli from the dead spaces. Then doubtless the remaining oxygen will provide a useful supplement to the depleted reserves in the blood prior to resurfacing. Clearly a large lung would not serve any useful purpose to any form in which the lung collapses during a substantial part of the dive except in so far as some of the contained gas could be utilized towards the end of a dive and it is not surprising therefore that it is only shallow-diving species which have relatively large lungs.

* Hydrostatic pressures are commonly given in terms of atmospheres, where 1 atmosphere is equivalent to 760 mm Hg or 101.325 kNm^{-2}, or in bars where 1 bar = 10^6 dynes cm^2 or 100 kNm^{-2} or 750.15 mm Hg at 0°C.

Porpoises have lungs a little larger than those of man at 6.6 l kg^{-1} body wt. (*Tursiops*) or 6.9 l kg^{-1} (*Phocoena*) and, since their dives are commonly fairly shallow, the lungs are likely to remain inflated except when they go deeper (cf. p. 24).

The sea otter, *Enhydra lutris*, also a shallow diver, seems to be one of the few marine species with a lung volume which is large relative to that of man (Fig. 2–1).

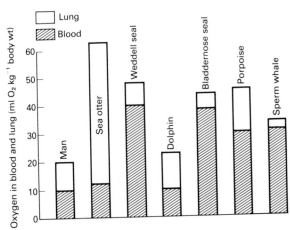

Fig. 2–1   Initial oxygen volumes in the blood and lungs of various species at the start of a dive.

2.2   Oxygen in blood

The maximum concentration of oxygen carried in solution in the blood of mammals breathing air at atmospheric pressure is about 0.3 ml per 100 ml blood. Total oxygen-carrying capacity of the blood in most vertebrates is very much higher than this due to the combination with the pigment haemoglobin in the red blood cells. Generally the overall capacity is some 50 to 100 times the amount carried in solution, the precise amount varying with the haematocrit (the percentage of blood volume occupied by red blood cells) and the concentration of haemoglobin per cell.

Animals exposed to continuous hypoxia (low availability of oxygen) as a result of living at high altitudes or in partially de-oxygenated waters generally have rather higher haematocrits than related forms which experience greater environmental oxygen levels. Such adjustments can also occur to some extent at the level of the individual, the haematocrit tending to increase, for example, in mountaineers who spend long periods at high altitude and also in fish maintained in low O_2 media.

Diving animals, though breathing air at atmospheric pressure, experience the problem of asphyxia during dives and, not surprisingly, they also tend to have high haematrocrit values so that the O_2 carrying capacity of the blood is also often rather above the average for vertebrates (Table 2).

Table 2

	Hb (g 100 ml^{-1} blood)	O_2 capacity (vol %)	Blood volume (ml kg^{-1} body wt.)	O_2 (ml kg^{-1} body wt.)
Man	16	20	80	16
Dog	14.8	21.8	86	18.7
Horse	11.1	21.4	62	13.3
Hen	10.3	14.0	90	12.6
Gentoo penguin	—	20.7	90	18.6
Duck (domestic)	14.8	17.0	102	17.3
Guillemot	—	26.0	137	35.6
Bottlenose dolphin	15.9	21.2	71	15.0
White sided dolphin	—	25.6	108	27.6
Porpoise (*Phocoena communis*)	—	20.5	150	30.7
Harbour seal	20.0	26.4	159	42.0
Weddell seal	—	35.5	—	40
Elephant seal	20.7	27.5	207	56.9
Pygmy sperm whale	15.7	32.4	—	—

The total capacity of the blood to store oxygen in the pre-dive state is further enhanced in diving mammals by the fact that they possess unusually large blood volumes relative to those of terrestrial species. Furthermore, the real difference in blood volume between divers and non-divers is perhaps even more marked in terms of volume per unit weight of metabolizing tissue than the figures in Table 2 suggest, since the inert blubber can form a substantial part of the body weight (up to 40%). For instance, correction of the figures to account for the fat load puts up the elephant seal blood volume value from 207 to 318 ml kg^{-1} whereas comparable adjustment for man (average rather than corpulent) increases the volume only from 80 to 96 ml kg^{-1}.

Enlarged blood volume increases the overall amount of oxygen carried in the blood but, in order to make effective use of the bound gas, the animals must also be able to unload it from combination with haemoglobin where it is required, i.e. at the tissue level.

Oxygen dissociates from haemoglobin as the partial pressure of O_2 in the surrounding medium drops (Fig. 2–2). The presence of CO_2 in the medium enhances this effect, so that at any given partial pressure of O_2 less oxygen can be bound to haemoglobin than in the absence of CO_2. This transference of the dissociation curve to the right in the presence of CO_2 is termed the *Bohr shift*. The larger the Bohr shift the greater is the tendency for oxygen to unload and hence the better the potential utilization of the bound O_2. Appropriate to their diving habit and the need to make maximal use of the O_2 carried down at the start of the dive, marine mammals tend to display a rather large Bohr shift in relation to that of most terrestrial species. In addition, at least the larger marine mammals also have haemoglobin with a fairly high half loading tension for oxygen ($P_{50}(O_2)$) (Table 3) so that at tissue partial pressure a large part of the bound oxygen is made available.

Table 3

Species	$P_{50}(O_2)$ mm Hg (at pH 7.4)	Bohr Effect
Divers		
Pacific white sided dolphin (*Lagenorhynchus*)	24.8	0.717
Bottle nose dolphin (*Tursiops*)	26.8	0.664
Pacific bottlenose (*Tursiops*)	26.0	0.712
Pilot whale (*Globicephala*)	31.2	0.622
Killer whale (*Orcinus*)	30.7	0.738
Risso dolphin (*Grampus*)	30.5	0.972
Sperm whale (*Physeter*)	26.5	0.478
Harbour seal (*Phoca*)	31.0	0.534
Elephant seal (*Mirounga*)	30.5	0.634
Non-divers		
Cow (*Bos*)	27.6	0.56
Goat (*Capra*)	30	0.53
Elephant (*Loxodonta*)	22.4	0.4
Dog (*Canis*)	28.3	0.57 → 0.48

One potential disadvantage of the possession of a large Bohr shift is that, if the CO_2 tension in the lung is high, the blood will not become fully saturated with oxygen during its passage through the respiratory organ. Marine mammals overcome this problem by evacuating the lungs more fully at each breath when at the surface than do most terrestrial species. Excess CO_2 accumulated during a dive can thus be rapidly removed from the lungs and blood so that the body fluid can be fully re-oxygenated once more.

One further factor may possibly contribute to the high oxygen capacity of the blood of some cetaceans. Analysis of the haemoglobin of the blood of the pygmy sperm whale and some related delphinids suggests that the oxygen-binding capacity exceeds the normal level of 1.38 ml O$_2$ g^{-1} haemoglobin which pertains in terrestrial forms. It is not yet clear whether such a high level of binding, (up to 2.07 ml O$_2$ g^{-1} Hb in the pygmy sperm whale) is due to the presence of more iron molecules per gram haemoglobin (since 1 molecule of oxygen is usually associated with 1 atom of iron) or whether some different type of oxygen-binding molecule is present.

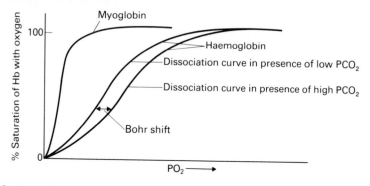

Fig. 2–2 Comparison of the dissociation curves for haemoglobin and myoglobin and the effect (Bohr shift) of increasing the PCO$_2$ on the oxygen binding capacity of haemoglobin.

The greater oxygen capacity per unit volume and large blood volume per unit weight of diving species can, in animals such as the bladdernose seal, increase the available oxygen within the blood at submergence by a factor of some two to four over that of equivalent sized land animals (Fig. 2–1).

2.3   Muscle O$_2$ levels

The muscles of diving species are generally darker in colour than those of terrestrial forms (some whale muscles appearing almost black) as a result of the large amount of the oxygen-binding pigment myoglobin present. Seal muscle can contain up to seven times the concentration of myoglobin found in the corresponding muscles of cattle and, as a result of the presence of this pigment, a considerable proportion of the overall oxygen present in the body of animals at the start of a dive is in the muscles. In seals nearly half of total oxygen present on submergence is in the form of oxymyoglobin and the oxygen content of individual muscles, on a weight basis, may reach one-fifth of that of the blood.

The affinity of myoglobin for oxygen is considerably greater than that for haemoglobin (Fig. 2–2) so that it requires markedly lower oxygen tensions before the oxygen can separate from the protein than is the case with haemoglobin. Consequently oxygen *cannot* be unloaded from myoglobin and pass to haemoglobin for re-distribution to other tissues. Oxygen in the muscles at the start of a dive can therefore only be utilized by that tissue.

2.4   Possible control of buoyancy as an aid to conservation of oxygen

The limited amount of oxygen present at the start of a dive necessitates the development of physiological and biochemical means of conservation for the benefit of the more oxygen sensitive tissues. These aspects will be discussed shortly, but first we may consider the obvious point that restriction of swimming activity will assist in prolonging a dive. In this respect CLARKE (1978) has recently presented some compelling evidence in support of a hypothesis that by adjusting the density of the spermaceti organs (Fig. 2–3) (which can constitute 7.5% of the weight of the whale)

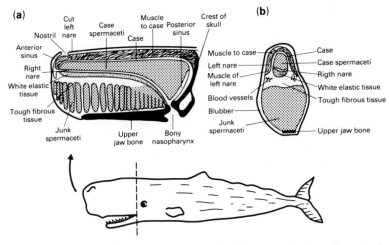

Fig. 2–3   Diagrammatic sections of the head of a sperm whale to illustrate, in (a) LS and (b) TS, the location of spermaceti. ((a) and (b) after CLARKE, M. R. (1970). *Nature, Lond.*, **228**, 873–74.)

the sperm whale may be able to attain near neutral buoyancy and so potentially be capable of maintaining position in the water at depth without the expenditure of much mechanical energy. The spermaceti organ could of course have other roles, including acting as a sonic lens in conjunction with the whale's echolocation system, but these could be compatible with the buoyancy function. Clarke shows that the density of spermaceti changes sufficiently with temperature to be potentially capable of effecting buoyancy control. Furthermore, the fact that there is a blood supply passing via the skin to the spermaceti and a possibility that the right nare may be used as a water-cooling channel suggests that the anatomy of the system is suitable for density changes to be effected by temperature adjustments. Proof that the spermaceti organ is used in this way remains to be obtained but additional pointers to the function of the spermaceti in some such fashion are (a) that diving sperm whales often emerge from a dive close to their point of submergence (which suggests that lateral swimming is restricted) and (b) that other deep, long-diving whales such as the bottlenose *Hyperoodon* and the pygmy sperm whale *Kogia* both have spermaceti oil in the snout. Whales such as the fin whale *Balaenoptera physalus* may occasionally dive to 500 m but only for periods of a few minutes. Furthermore, the fin whale tends to cover a considerable lateral distance when diving, implying that it swims continuously throughout the period of submergence. Doubtless this vigorous activity restricts the length of dive.

The concept that sperm whales may be relatively inactive once at depth would be compatible with an old hypothesis erected to offer an explanation for the fact that the tall conical teeth of the whale are present only in the lower jaw. The theory holds that bioluminescent squid swim to investigate the reflection of their own light from the polished surface of the teeth as the whale moves slowly along with its mouth open!

Some possible support for the view that the whale may swim near the bottom with the mouth open comes from the finding that sperm whales which have become entangled in submarine cables almost invariably seem to have had the cable caught in the mouth prior to secondary entanglements around the fins and flukes. Further evidence is needed, however, before such ideas can be accepted unequivocably, attractive though they be.

3 Metabolic Responses to Diving

Examination of the muscle O_2 level during submergence of seals shows that the oxygen reserves are rapidly utilized and that virtually none remains after five minutes apnoea even though the blood oxygen level has only declined by some 14% at this time (Fig. 3–1).

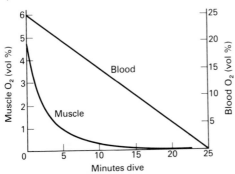

Fig. 3–1 Relative rates of decrease in the oxygen content of muscle and blood in the harbour seal (*Phoca vitulina*) during a dive. (After SCHOLANDER, P. F., IRVING, L. and GRINNELL, S. W. (1942). *J. biol. Chem.*, **142**, 431.)

It is clear, therefore, that prolongation of dives beyond some five minutes cannot be dependent upon continued utilization of muscle oxygen reserves. Furthermore, lung and blood oxygen also are insufficient to last for the known periods of dives even if only the resting metabolic rates shown by the animals at the surface pertain during submergence (Table 4). It would therefore be necessary to postulate some

Table 4 (Data from ANDERSEN, 1966 and CLARKE, 1978.)

Animal	Available O_2(ml) in lung, blood and muscle	Resting metabolic rate (ml O_2 min^{-1})	Est. dive time (min)	Actual dive time (max) (min)
Duck	85	22	4	15
Penguin	270	100	3	7
Seal	1520	250	6	18
Porpoise	1090	450	3	
Fin whale	3 350 l.	200 l.	17	30
Bottlenose	109 l.	3–4000	36	120
Sperm whale	1 735 l.	49 l.	35	75

other explanation of prolonged dives than increase in stored oxygen, even if the animals remained quiescent under water. In fact, as is obvious, they swim actively and consequently expend more energy than in the resting state.

Resolution of the apparent paradox could be achieved if the animals either (a) build up a large oxygen debt while submerged which is then repaid when air breathing is resumed, or (b) utilize oxygen at a lower rate when submerged than at the surface. As is usually the case in biological systems where two solutions to a problem are possible, both are utilized to varying degrees by different species.

3.1   Oxygen debt

Once the oxygen initially in the muscle has been used up, the tissue is dependent primarily upon glycolysis for its source of energy, since most muscles are deprived of a blood supply during a dive. Glycolysis in the absence of oxygen leads to the production of lactic and other organic acids which are largely stored in the muscle tissues until the termination of the dive, though in both diving birds and seals some lactate may escape into the blood towards the end of a long dive. In reptiles such as the turtle *Pseudemys scripta*, the lactic acid levels in the venous blood can rise from some 3.6 mmol l^{-1} in air-breathing controls to the astonishingly high level of 50 mmol l^{-1} after a dive lasting 24 hours and even to 60 mmol l^{-1} after 24 hours in N_2. These values may be compared with the peak lactate levels in the blood of seals on surfacing of some 20 mmol l^{-1} and the maximum level in man after violent exercise of some 10–20 mmol l^{-1}.

Unlike the situation in birds and mammals, in the turtle the central nervous system is able to derive its metabolic energy almost totally from anaerobic metabolism. Glycolysis is necessary for the supply of energy to the brain during the dive and if metabolism is blocked turtles rapidly succumb.

Increasing lactic acid levels in the blood cause a decline in blood pH, though bicarbonate and other buffers limit the extent of the change. Decline in pH produces a consequent increase in the partial pressure of CO_2 in the blood. In man the respiratory centre is rather sensitive to raised CO_2 pressure and, when this occurs, initiates an increase in the respiratory rates. Similarly, if air with a high CO_2 level is breathed, the respiratory rate rises (Fig. 3–2). The seal, appropriately, is much less sensitive to CO_2 and presumably this is a factor enabling it to prolong apnoea.

Marine diving forms also tend to have both a greater buffering reserve in the blood and, because they have more haemoglobin, a larger capacity to mop up excess CO_2 in the form of carbamino-haemoglobin. Both these features will also serve to delay arrival at the critical CO_2 level which forces re-surfacing. Some prolongation of breath-holding dives by man

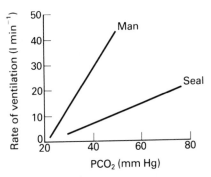

Fig. 3–2 Comparison of the rate of lung ventilation in man and seal in relation to blood CO_2 levels. (Adapted from ROBIN, E. D. (1966) and reprinted, by permission, from *New England J. Medicine*, **275**, 646–52.)

can be achieved if the subject hyperventilates beforehand to lower the CO_2 level in the lung below normal and so allow a longer period before CO_2 builds up to stress levels during apnoea. Interestingly, a dolphin (*Tursiops*) which had been trained to dive on command also tended to hyperventilate when anticipating a deep dive and pochard ducks double the respiratory rate shortly before natural dives.

In man, a build up of CO_2 in the blood eventually forces breathing to be re-initiated during voluntary apnoea – a point well illustrated by the fact that men who die of asphyxia at sea invariably have water in the lungs.

One factor which contributes to the ability of marine mammals to dive for extended periods is that the stimulus to surface in order to breathe can be resisted longer in the diving form because in at least some cetaceans the control of respiration has effectively passed from the involuntary centres in the medulla to the voluntary centres in the cortex. Indeed one of the problems of operating on a dolphin is that it stops breathing when rendered unconscious by anaesthetic. Sleep in these animals (*Tursiops*) might thus appear to present a potential hazard but it is reported that they almost invariably sleep with one eye open and one closed so that presumably half the sensory inputs are always operating. Each eye has two to three hours of sleep per day.

3.2 Metabolic rate

For a wide range of size in warm-blooded animals the metabolic rate, or oxygen consumption, varies as $KW^{0.73}$ where K is a constant and W is the body weight. Most animals in the range of size from mouse to elephant therefore lie on a straight line when a double logarithmic plot of body weight against calorific output is constructed. However, marine mammals tend to form an exception to the general rule having metabolic rates averaging some 1.5–2 times that to be expected from their weight. Although this finding lends no support to the concept that the overall metabolism of these animals might be depressed below that of terrestrial forms, evidence is forthcoming from work on seals which suggests that during the course of a passive dive (i.e. with the animal restrained) the metabolic rate may fall to about one quarter of that when the animal is breathing air at the surface. This conclusion is based on the fact that the oxygen debt, which is built up during a dive and repaid subsequently by excess oxygen consumption, represents only about 25% of that expected from the length of dive if the metabolic rate had been normal. Birds too show a similar drop in metabolic rate on diving; indeed, the temperature of a duck begins to fall even if only its head is immersed in water.

Such a drop in metabolic rate tends to conserve the oxygen stores in the blood. In turtles, by contrast, decline in heat production and blood oxygen levels are contemporaneous suggesting that general tissue asphyxia is the cause of decreased metabolic rates (Fig. 3–3).

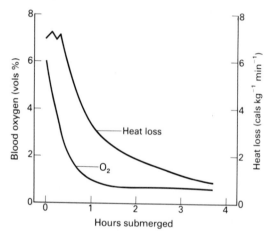

Fig. 3–3   Decline in metabolic rate and blood oxygen level in the turtle (*Pseudemys scripta*) during diving. (Much modified after JACKSON, D. C. (1968). *J. appl. Physiol.*, **24**, 503.) (1 cal = 4.186 J.)

However, there are parallels between the effect in the turtle and the warm-blooded forms in so far as the oxygen conserving mechanism in the latter operates by depriving non-vital tissues of blood and it is the state of asphyxia of these ischaemic tissues which decreases the overall metabolic rate.

4 Cardiovascular Responses

4.1 Peripheral resistance

Calculations based on the cardiac output of the grey seal (*Halichoerus*) prior to and during a dive suggest that the resistance to the flow of blood in the peripheral parts of the circulatory system increases some twelve-fold soon after submergence. This increase in peripheral resistance arises as a result of constriction of the smooth muscle in the walls of arteries and arterioles under the influence of the sympathetic vasomotor nerve supply to the blood vessels.

Not all tissues are affected equally. The voluntary muscles (with the exception of the jaw and eye muscles) and many of the viscera, including the stomach, virtually lose their blood supply (Table 5) in both mammals

Table 5 Reduction in blood flow through muscle and visceral tissues of a seal during a dive. Flow is given in ml 100 g tissue^{-1} min^{-1}. Note large reduction in kidney, muscle and stomach blood flow and smaller percentage reduction in cerebral flow. Note also the reduction in heart rate but relative constancy of blood pressure. (Simplified from BLIX, A. S., KJEKSHUS, J. K., ENGE, I. and BERGEN, A. (1976). *Acta physiol. skand.*, **96**, 277.)

	Control	Diving Animal
Muscle (*M. psoas*)	14	0
Kidney	135	3
Stomach	14	0
Cerebrum	143	49
Heart rate (BPM)	132	10
Blood pressure (mm Hg)	165	155

and birds. Filtration in the kidneys stops during the dive so urine production ceases. As a result of this cessation of blood supply, any damage to the affected areas results in very little bleeding during a dive though profuse blood loss on surfacing indicates the return of blood supply.

When an X-ray opaque material is injected into the aortic arch and its passage is followed by radiography, it is observed that the material rapidly disappears from the main arteries in seals (*Phoca vitulina*) which are at the surface, but that it is removed only slowly in diving individuals. X-ray pictures suggest that the main arteries supplying the body regions posterior to the heart constrict close to their origin from the aorta. Furthermore, the X-ray records are similar in appearance irrespective of the time interval after the start of the dive. It seems likely therefore that, at least on a gross scale, the constriction of the arteries persists throughout the dive. Whether or not it is possible during an extended dive for some temporary relaxation on a local level to restore blood supply to regions suffering severely from lack of metabolites or oxygen remains unresolved.

By contrast with the situation in the posterior part of the body, the blood supply of the head is much less affected during a dive. In ducks the masseter (jaw adductor) muscle receives a normal supply and so too do the eye muscles, oesophagus and brain. Such a distribution doubtless reflects the need for peak sensory and motor responses in the search for and swallowing of food.

If one may judge from experiments where radioactive rubidium is injected into the blood stream and its rate of uptake into different tissues is measured in diving and surface individuals, then there is some evidence that the blood flow to certain glands, including the adrenals and thyroid, can increase during a dive.

Restriction of the blood circulation to certain tissues naturally limits the rate of oxygen utilization and conserves the oxygen in the blood for those organs such as the heart and brain which are oxygen demanding. The value of this feature in prolonging the dive can readily be illustrated by measurement of oxygen utilization in *Phoca vitulina*. When the seal is at the surface the animal utilizes oxygen at a rate of some 250 ml min^{-1} of which the brain requires some 50 ml min^{-1}. Restriction of the circulation to other tissues should therefore potentially extend the period of a dive some five-fold. Appropriate to this argument is the observation that whereas a seal can normally dive for 15–20 min its limit is only about 4 min after treatment with sufficient atropine to block the vasomotor nerves to the arteries and so prevent the increase in the peripheral resistance.

Sudden cessation of blood flow through peripheral tissues might be expected to result in venous blood flow being sluggish in the affected parts of the body. Since the venous blood, at least at the start of a dive, will still have a relatively high oxygen content it would be anticipated *a priori* that mechanisms would be developed to ensure that this blood is returned to the central circulation so that its oxygen could be utilized by the more sensitive tissues. Special blood vessels which form direct arteriovenous shunts in the web of the feet of diving birds and seals could have this function. By short-circuiting the capillary beds these vessels permit such blood flow as there is in the leg arteries to be used to 'flush through' the venous blood without appreciable loss of oxygen to the tissues during the passage of blood through the shunt.

Curtailing the blood supply to those tissues which do not suffer impairment following temporary oxygen lack has the secondary consequence that waste metabolites from the tissues cannot be released into the circulation until blood flow returns to normal at the termination of the dive.

Consequently, on surfacing there is a sudden flow of lactic acid into the blood as circulation is restored to the muscles (Fig. 4–1).

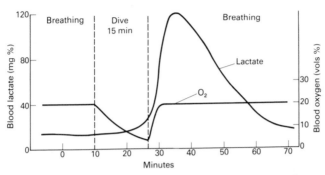

Fig. 4–1   Lactic acid levels in the blood of a seal during diving and post-dive recovery. Note that blood lactic acid levels scarcely increase during a dive but rise sharply when the animal surfaces. (Modified after SCHOLANDER, 1962.)

4.2   Bradycardia (slowing of the heart rate)

If both the heart rate and volume of fluid expelled from the heart per beat (stroke volume) remained at normal levels during a dive despite the increase in peripheral resistance, the blood pressure would rise substantially. No such increase in pressure occurs because, in most diving forms, although the stroke volume appears to be relatively unchanged, the heart rate and, therefore, overall cardiac output tend to drop sharply during submergence. Conversely, on emergence, heart rate and cardiac output increase initially to levels greater than the pre-dive rates and then gradually revert to normal.

Such effects are well illustrated by the domestic duck *Anas boscas*. At rest the average heart rate is 244 beats min^{-1} and the cardiac output some 1500 ml min^{-1}. Within 2 min of forced submergence both factors decrease some twenty-fold but within 1–2 s of surfacing again there is a rapid increase in heart rate to 300–500 beats min^{-1} attended by a rise in arterial pressure. Accompanying this tachycardia on surfacing, vasodilatation occurs and cardiac output rises briefly to 2500–4000 ml min^{-1}. Both heart rate and cardiac output then decline to the pre-dive levels over about 6–8 min.

Comparable effects on both submergence and surfacing occur in a wide range of diving mammals and birds (Fig. 4–2).

An analogous bradycardial response to changed respiratory conditions may also be observed in species of fish (though not in the hagfish

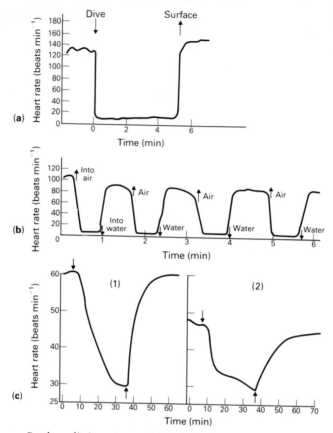

Fig. 4–2 Bradycardia in various animals. (a) In the harbour seal during a forced dive. (After ELSNER, R. (1965). *Hvalradets Skrifter*, **48**, 24.) (b) In the grunion (*Leuresthes*) on removing the fish from the water. (After GAREY, W. F. (1962). *Biol. Bull.*, **122**, 362.) (c) In the frog (*Rana temporaria*) (1) before and (2) after bilateral vagotomy. (After JONES, D. and SHELTON, G. (1964). *J. exp. Biol.*, **41**, 417.) Arrows indicate time of submergence and emergence.

(*Agnatha*), which lacks cardioregulatory nerves). The grunion (*Leuresthes*), a small pelagic fish living off the Californian coast, has the curious habit of laying its eggs at the extreme high water level reached on spring tides. Males and females wriggle to the limit of the waves, the eggs are laid and fertilized and then the fish retreat offshore; bradycardia occurs in this fish when it is taken out of water (Fig. 4–2b) and presumably will also occur in breeding migrations up the beach. Cod and the flying fish *Cypselurus* also show slowing of the heart rhythm when removed from water.

Conversely the Australian fish (*Periophthalmodon australis*) (mudskipper), which spends much of its time on exposed mud flats, shows a normal heartbeat when in air but a reduced rate when it retreats into its burrows. This finding may at first appear paradoxical until it is appreciated that the burrows are normally filled with stagnant water. Consequently, the probable explanation of its behaviour is that the heart rate changes are initiated centrally in response to asphyxia. Such asphyxial responses due to hypercapnia (excess CO_2 in the blood) or hypoxia (too little O_2) also play their part in the development of the full diving bradycardia in higher forms though emotional and reflex responses are also involved. Consideration of the responses of a range of animals will perhaps illustrate the point. In the frog (Rana temporaria) two types of bradycardia can occur. One is a gradual slowing of the heart over a period of some 15–30 min after submergence (Fig 4–2c). Such a response is primarily due to a direct effect of asphyxia on the heart since prior section of the vagus nerve (stimulation of which will slow the heart) has no effect on the development of bradycardia. The other is a more rapid onset of bradycardia over 1 min initiated by the central nervous system and mediated via the vagus nerve.

Alligators have an interesting response in so far as bradycardia is not observed if the animal is left to itself to dive but if it is disturbed during the dive – as by the approaching footsteps of the experimenter – bradycardia immediately occurs. One interpretation of this response is that bradycardia in the disturbed animal will, in conjunction with increased peripheral resistance, reduce its rate of oxygen consumption and so enable it to prolong its dive.

In seals also there seems to be a psychological component since bradycardia does not always develop if the animal is sufficiently close to the surface that it can reach up and breathe if it wishes, though normally when it dives bradycardia occurs within a few seconds. Furthermore, when seals dive naturally the onset of bradycardia is slightly slower than when they are agitated by being strapped to a board prior to artificial submergence (Fig. 4–2a) though in both cases the pulse rate will ultimately drop to some 10% of the surface value. One respiratory physiologist claims that the agitation of seals about to undergo diving experiments may be dispelled if music is played to them and that the music of Bach has a more effective calming influence than that of the Beatles!

Bradycardia occurs in man, especially in those accustomed to diving, though it is less pronounced than in specialist diving species. Rats, too, show moderately well developed bradycardia after submergence. Taking into account the comparable response in fish and reptiles it would seem, therefore, that bradycardia is a very ancient physiological feature of the vertebrate line.

4.2.1   Initiation of bradycardia

Both stimulation of the face, particularly around the nostrils, and absence of the chest movements which normally accompany breathing are probably implicated in initiating bradycardia and other diving responses. In man cessation of respiratory movements alone, as in breath-holding in air, causes little or no bradycardia though immersion of the face in water, particularly cold water, results in both slowing of the heart and decrease in flow of blood in the forearm. Merely holding a duck or cormorant with its head down can result in cessation of breathing and heart slowing, the so-called postural apnoea. In the duck development of full bradycardia has two phases: (1) a rapid but relatively modest retardation of heart beat to some 60–70% of the pre-dive level, immediately after the forced immersion of the head, and (2) a more gradual intensification of heart slowing starting some 15–20 s after the commencement of the dive (Fig. 4–3). In a dive the full extent of

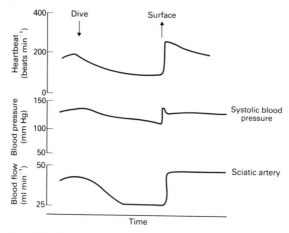

Fig. 4–3 Modifications of the heart rate, systolic blood pressure and sciatic artery blood flow in a domestic duck (*Anas boscas*) diving. Note the relative constancy of blood pressure despite the substantial changes in heart rate and blood flow. (After BUTLER, P. J. and JONES, D. (1971). *J. Physiol., Lond.*, **214**, 457–79.)

bradycardia is evident within 60 s and the heart rate then is some 10–15 beats min⁻¹ by comparison with initial values around 200. However, if the air sacs are perfused with oxygen while the bird is under water, only the initial rapid phase of heart beat slowing occurs, the rate dropping to about 150 beats min⁻¹. Also in these latter circumstances, the increase in peripheral resistance is less pronounced. These findings have been interpreted as indicating that facial stimulation and apnoea are responsible for the initial response and that the secondary slowing occurs as a reflex in response to blood gas changes. Support for this conclusion is given by observations that when birds fail to exhale before diving, bradycardia is delayed. Probably the response to lowered arterial O_2 and increased CO_2 are initiated by the chemoreceptors of the carotid body, since if the carotid sinus and aortic nerve are sectioned, the vaso-constrictor response causing increased peripheral resistance is intensified if hypercapnia (excess CO_2) is superimposed on hypoxia.

Closure of the nostrils of seals in air results in the onset of bradycardia very similar to that of ducks, heart rate falling gradually from 130 to 15 beats min^{-1} in 48 s. Slow onset of bradycardia in such a manner suggests that an asphyxial response can occur also in these mammals. Such a conclusion seems to be supported by the observation that if respiratory movements are maintained in submerged seals by provision of an air supply, and if the facial nerves are at the same time rendered insensitive by the application of a local anaesthetic, no bradycardia is observed. However, sudden forced immersion of a seal into water results in a much faster onset of bradycardia than merely closing the nostrils in air, the heart rate falling virtually instantaneously to less than 20 beats min^{-1} (Fig. 4–3). Such a response suggests that, in the mammal, maximal bradycardia can be initiated by psychological effects even before 'asphyxial' changes in the blood gases come into play.

In summary therefore it seems that bradycardia can be initiated either by the effect of direct anoxia on the heart (as in vagally denervated frogs) or via the cardio-inhibiting activity of the vagus nerve. Vagal inhibition may be generated by emotional response, by reflex response to cessation of respiratory movements and by the wetting of the nostril area or by reflex chemosensory response to increasing hypercapnia and hypoxia.

In view of man's interest in diving on his own account there has been intensive study of the reflexes associated with submergence in terrestrial mammals and in some respect indeed more is known of their responses than of those of natural diving species. In general, there is a qualitative similarity between the reflexes of both diving and terrestrial species as indicated by the summary of findings on terrestrial species given by ANGELL JAMES and DE BURGH DALY (1972). They suggest:

1. Immersion of the head initiates a reflex acting via the 5th cranial nerve which results in cessation of breathing and stimulation of cardio-inhibitory and vaso-motor centres in the brain. These centres in turn cause bradycardia and vasoconstriction in the skin, muscles, intestines and kidney.

2. The lack of stimulation from stretch receptors in the partially collapsed lung during apnoea enhances the effect in (1) but conversely activity in lung receptors produced by inflating the lung can override the primary reflex responses.

3. Activity in the expiratory centre in the brain further reinforces the cardio-inhibitory response mediated by the vagus nerve.

4. As hypoxia and hypercapnia develop, peripheral arterial chemo-receptors initiate further stimulation of the cardio-inhibitory and vasomotor responses. The carotid bodies, a principal source of chemo-

sensory response to blood gas changes, excite the respiratory centre to initiate breathing but this effect is overridden by the trigeminal (5th cranial nerve) reflex during short dives.

5. Reflex activation of the sympathetic system involves stimulation of the suprarenal medulla and release of catechol amines (adrenalin and non-adrenalin) as well as vasoconstriction. The catechol amines may in turn modify the chemoreceptor response of the carotid bodies and potentiate the constriction of peripheral blood vessels (Fig. 4.4).

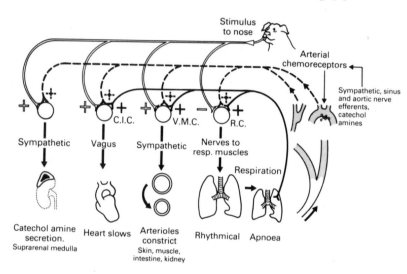

Fig. 4–4 Diagrammatic representation of proposed sequence of events occurring in mammals during submersion. Stimulation by water of trigeminal nerve receptors in and around the nose and on the face leads to reflex apnoea in the expiratory position, bradycardia, vasoconstriction and secretion of suprarenal catecholamines (*open lines*). The apnoea in turn causes a reduction in activity of a pulmonary vagal reflex resulting in bradycardia and vaso-constriction (*solid lines*). Then arterial hypoxia and hypercapnia stimulate the arterial chemoreceptors which reflexly reinforce the cardio-inhibitory, vaso-constrictor and humoral responses (*interrupted lines*). C.I.C., cardio-inhibitory centre; V.M.C., vasomotor centre; R.C., respiratory centres. +, stimulation; –, inhibition. (From ANGELL JAMES and DE BURGH DALY (1972).)

4.3 Origins of diving responses

As far as the mammals are concerned, it is not surprising that heart slowing and increased peripheral resistance in response to asphyxial conditions are so widespread, since mammals universally experience such a syndrome at birth. Appropriately, young mammals, including human offspring, then show marked bradycardia until the first breath is taken and thereafter, as in a surfacing seal, there is a flood of lactic acid into the blood indicating that vaso-constriction had accompanied the heart slowing during the period of oxygen deprivation which accompanies the birth process.

5 Biochemical Adaptations

The progressive hypoxia which air-breathing forms experience during a dive is reflected in various modifications to the enzyme systems involved in metabolism. Two enzymes in particular, lactic dehydrogenase and pyruvic kinase, are known to show some correlation with diving capability.

5.1 Role of lactate dehydrogenase

Lactate dehydrogenase (LDH) which catalyses the reaction

$$\underset{\text{(pyruvate)}}{CH_3 COCO_2^- + NADH + H^+} \quad \overset{LDH}{\rightleftharpoons} \quad \underset{\text{(lactate)}}{CH_3 CHOHCO_2^- + NAD^+}$$

is a tetramer, i.e. it is composed of four protein sub-units acting in conjunction. These proteins are of two types, H which primarily catalyses the reaction lactate to pyruvate and the M type which is principally concerned with the reverse reaction. Five possible combinations of H and M occur: H_4, H_3M, H_2M_2, HM_3 and M_4. In terrestrial animals the H_4 type predominates in the essentially aerobic tissues, heart and brain, while the M_4 type dominates in skeletal muscle (cf. sheep in Table 6) in which high

Table 6   Isozyme type as % total LDH. (Slightly modified from BLIX, A. S. (1971). *Comp. Biochem. Physiol.*, **40B**, 579.)

	H_4	H_3M	H_2M_2	HM_3	M_4
Seal					
Brain	29 ± 8	40 ± 7	23 ± 6	5 ± 3	3 ± 4
Heart	33 ± 5	49 ± 5	12 ± 5	4 ± 2	2 ± 4
Skeletal muscle	2 ± 2	10 ± 8	23 ± 4	29 ± 4	36 ± 11
Sheep					
Brain	39 ± 4	21 ± 1	36 ± 1	4 ± 3	—
Heart	88 ± 8	12 ± 7	—	—	—
Skeletal muscle	4 ± 4	5 ± 3	5 ± 2	4 ± 4	82 ± 9

lactate levels can be built up during activity. By contrast, in a diving form such as the seal, where the central nervous system is perforce likely to experience some lowering of oxygen tension in the blood towards the end of a dive, the brain LDH contains a higher proportion of M-containing isozymes. This factor, coupled with the observation that the Weddell seal brain contains some two to three times as much glycogen as does that of terrestrial forms, suggests that cerebral tissues in this species may be adapted to tolerate some measure of anaerobiosis during submersion, whereas the brain cells of land animals tend to be extremely intolerant of O_2 lack. Confirmation that a measure of relative anaerobiosis may indeed be tolerated for a time by the seal brain comes from experiments in which electroencephalograph studies were combined with measurements of the oxygen and lactic acid levels in the blood entering and leaving the cranium. During about the last quarter of a dive the rate of oxygen extraction by the brain from the oxygen-depleted blood begins to decline and lactate is added to the blood within the cranium. However, electroencephalograms show no indication of stress until the arterial oxygen level has fallen to about 10 mm Hg which is only some 20% of the arterial O_2 pressure when the blood is in equilibrium with atmospheric O_2 in the lungs at the surface. The presence of additional lactate in the blood implies that the seal brain can obtain some of its energy from anaerobic metabolism, a feature unknown in terrestrial mammals.

The percentage of M-containing isozymes in the heart of whales is even more striking than in the seal (humpback 17%, fin 20%, sei 20% and sperm whale 45%) and it is also noteworthy that it is the deep-diving sperm whale which contains the highest levels. The total LDH is higher in the sperm whale than in the baleen whales which seems appropriate in view of the latter's generally shorter and shallower dives.

Variation in the isozyme distribution between diving and non-diving species are also known from among bird, turtle and frog species. The eider duck is particularly curious in so far as from embryo to adult it only possesses the M_4 isozyme.

Pseudemys scripta, by mammalian standards, shows a truly remarkable ability to tolerate O_2 lack since the animal can remain submerged for several days, survive 100% N_2 for many hours and even tolerate injections of cyanide of some 10 times the level which would kill man – all without apparent permanent ill-effect.

During a dive the oxygen levels in a turtle's blood fall rapidly and after 48 h the ppO_2 is down to 0–2 mm Hg so there is no question but that the brain tolerates low O_2 levels and must be capable of obtaining its energy by anaerobic means to an even greater extent than the seal.

5.2   Role of pyruvate kinase

Pyruvate kinase, which catalyses the reaction phosphoenol pyruvate to pyruvate essentially unidirectionally provides a good measure of the potential rate of glycolysis in a tissue.

A positive correlation between the maximum dive time and pyruvate kinase levels has been shown in some diving forms (Table 7), suggesting that increased glycolysis may be involved in providing energy in long

Table 7   Maximum dive time and pyruvate kinase activity as μM conversion of phosphoenol pyruvate to pyruvate min^{-1} mg tissue protein^{-1}. (Values for sea lion and seals from SIMON, L. M. *et al.* (1974). *Comp. Biochem. Physiol.*, **47B**, 209. Values for rabbit from SIMON, L. M. and ROBIN, E. D. (1972). *Int. J. Biochem.*, **3**, 329.)

	Max. dive time (min)	Heart	Brain	Skeletal muscle
Sea lion (*Zalophus californianus*)	8	140	164	269
Harbour seal (*Phoca vitulina*)	20	174	262	562
Weddell seal (*Leptonychotes weddelli*)	60	386	302	565
Rabbit (*Oryctolagus (Lepus) curiculus*)	—	191	252	968

dives. Too much should not as yet be read into the limited number of results currently available, however, since the rabbit shows levels intermediate between two species of seal! The pyruvate kinase of the dolphin *Lagenorhynchus* is unusually sensitive to ATP levels, perhaps implying that, as ATP levels rise on the resumption of aerobic metabolism after a dive, pyruvate kinase is turned off thus sparing glucose at the expense of alternative metabolites such as fatty acids.

6 Anatomical Modifications

6.1 Modifications at the tissue and organ level

The increase of hydrostatic pressure with depth potentially creates two problems for animals which descend deeply: (1) risk of rupture damage to gas-filled spaces as the external pressure increases, and (2) increased rate of nitrogen entry into the blood as the partial pressure of N_2 in the lung is raised by compression of the contained air. If substantial uptake of nitrogen occurs there is a risk that on release of pressure, as an animal re-surfaces, bubbles of gas will appear in the blood and tissues causing disruption of circulation and other effects. Such bubble formation is of course the cause of the painful and dangerous syndrome which in man is known as 'caisson sickness' or 'bends' (cf. p. 49).

A number of anatomical modifications in marine mammals contribute to avoidance of damage from such causes: (1) the flexibility of the lung; (2) absence of connections between the thoracic wall and the lungs; (3) strengthening of the main airways with cartilage; (4) flexibility of the chest wall; (5) development of the retia mirabilia lining sinuses and within the thoracic region. To this list might be added reduction or loss of sinuses in the skull, other than those associated with the middle ear.

On diving to 200 m (660 ft) an animal would be expected to experience a decrease in volume of the gas in the lungs to about 5% of the initial volume, assuming no resistance of pressure by the chest wall. Inability of the lung to collapse to the extent required by this volume change would result in lesions and appropriately the lungs of diving species tend to be extremely flexible. They also lack connections to the thoracic wall so that the lung can, to some extent, collapse independently of the chest. By contrast the lungs of an elephant have extensive connections and the results of such an animal being forced to dive to 200 m would undoubtedly be lethal!

Partial collapse of the chest has been observed in man undertaking deep dives and underwater television pictures of the dolphin *Tursiops truncatus* at 300 m (1000 ft) show a comparable caving in of the thoracic region. Such caving without rupture of ribs is doubtless assisted by the fact that rib attachment is reduced in the cetacea to one (Mysticeti) or four or five (Odontoceti) articulations with the sternum. In the pygmy right whale (*Neobalæna*) all but the first three or four ribs have lost links with the vertebrae themselves. However, despite these modifications, collapse of the chest to match completely the decrease in the gas volume of the lungs is not required during a dive due to (1) the engorgement of the lung itself with blood and (2) the development in the thoracic region of an extensive plexi of blood vessels, the rete mirabile. Expansion of the rete with blood during a dive partially compensates for the volume change as the lung collapses. Interestingly the thoracic rete receive their blood supply from the posterior thoracic and intercostal arteries leaving the descending aorta and so can be filled relatively quickly when diving occurs. Similar retia mirabilia line the sinuses of the head thus limiting the risk of skull collapse at depth. These remarkable modifications to the blood system were extolled as long ago as 1680 by Tyson who reported that in cetaceans 'There is scarce any animal in which the veines and arteries are more curiously branched or more numerous than in this – they form a curious net-work and afford a very pleasant sight.'

Direct evidence of the forcing of the gases into the dead space during the dive comes from experiments in which a dolphin 'Tuffy' was trained by S. M. Ridgway's group to dive to a sonar beacon placed at various depths and then to ascend and breathe out into a container before finally surfacing. Analysis of the expired air showed that for dives of equal length *less* oxygen was utilized if the dive was deep than if it was shallow (Fig. 6–1), implying, of course, that the gas was not available to the respiratory surfaces during the whole period of a deep dive.

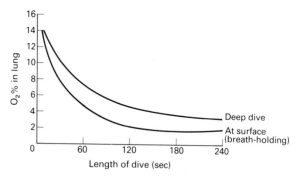

Fig. 6–1 Oxygen utilization from the lung of the dolphin (*Tursiops*) during shallow and deep dives to show that less oxygen is used in the deep dive. (After RIDGWAY, S. M., SCRONCE, B. L. and KANWISHER, J. (1969). *Science*, **166**, 1652. Copyright 1969 by the American Association for the Advancement of Science.)

Exclusion of gas from the lungs also restricts the penetration of nitrogen into the blood, as G. L. Kooyman has confirmed on the Weddell seal, and so limits the risk of bends. The possibility of bubble formation in vital areas in diving mammals is further lessened by the large amounts of fat present in the body. Nitrogen is preferentially soluble in fat and so will tend to some extent to be accommodated in lipid bodies rather than in more crucial areas. The effectiveness of nitrogen absorption into fat on a whole body basis is probably diminished by the lack of blood supply to fat-bearing tissues during diving but a considerable amount of a fatty foam is present in the sinuses and other air spaces of divers which may also help to absorb a proportion of the excess N_2.

As far as seals are concerned possible problems associated with N_2 absorption are further diminished by exhalation prior to diving which thus limits the amount of gas available. Penguins dive with a larger gas volume relative to body weight than any of the mammals (except the sea otter) and, at least in the gentoo and adelie penguins, 2 min dives (in a compression chamber) at 7.8 ATA result in rapid increase of blood nitrogen. Why such levels seem to produce neither nitrogen narcosis (raptures of the deep) at depth nor bends on surfacing is not clear at present. Presumably the sea otter never dives sufficiently deep for compression of lung gases to present a problem.

Volume and pressure changes in the throat and middle ear region pose a potential threat to the effective operation of the blood supply to and from the brain if this were to remain, as in terrestrial forms, primarily via the carotid artery and jugular vein. The internal carotid artery is still present in the pilot whale (*Globicephala*) and porpoise (*Phocaena*), it is atrophied in adult *Tursiops*. The role of the carotid is taken over in the latter by two large vessels in the spinal retial complex which have been termed spinal meningeal arteries though they are not strictly homologous with the meningeal arteries of terrestrial vertebrates. The dolphin vessels are intradural channels (and hence protected from pressure occlusion by the vertebral column) which pass over the cerebellum and then, after branching repeatedly, regroup near the pituitary, forming another retial complex before supplying the brain.

The function of the retial system in association with the brain supply is uncertain but may be involved in ensuring a continuous non-pulsating flow of blood to the central nervous system when the heart rate falls to only a few beats per minute.

In man and most other terrestrial forms there are two vertebral veins lying below the nerve cord. In seals these are replaced by a single dorsal extradural vein. As the jugular system is small it seems likely that this vein, also of course protected by the spinal column, has taken over the principal function of venous return from the cranium. The vessel sends down branches which supply the complex stellate plexus around the kidney. Whether or not this curious anatomical modification is designed to ensure that the cortex of the kidney does not suffer complete oxygen starvation during a dive, despite the cessation of the arterial supply noted earlier, remains to be established.

6.2   Cellular effects of high pressure

Raised pressures can produce a number of deleterious effects at the cellular level through modification of the sol-gel balance of protein systems, membrane structure and enzyme function.

Alteration of the sol-gel balance causes disturbance of amoeboid movement, pinocytosis, the activity of cilia and flagella, cleavage furrow initiation and mitotic spindle formation in dividing cells. Many of these syndromes are shown by the cells of normally surface-dwelling animals when they are suddenly exposed to pressures within or close to those experienced by the sperm whale on a 2000 m (6560 ft) dive. Thus 200 ATM blocks pinocytosis ('cell drinking') by *Amoeba* and also results in the production of abnormal pseudopodia. At a somewhat higher level (300 ATM) ciliary movement is affected in *Paramecium* and spindle formation and cell division cease in sea urchin eggs. The axonemes which support the relatively rigid axopoda of *Actinosphaerium* collapse at about the same order of pressure. All these effects can be ascribed to solation of microtubules.

The transport capabilities and permeability of membranes are affected by pressures of the order of 250–300 ATM. Frog nerves become hyperexcitable at this level and the muscles of the jellyfish *Cyanea* contract more frequently.

The activity of a number of enzymes may be influenced by pressures of about 200–300 atmospheres though many require much higher levels before being affected. Sensitive enzymes include Na-K-ATPase (this is involved in sodium transport) and succinic dehydrogenase (from *E. coli*). Both of these begin to show reduced activity at about 200 ATM.

Doubtless such effects contribute to the fact that a number of fish and invertebrates subsequently die if exposed to high pressures for short periods. Shrimps are reversibly immobilized by 200 ATM except for the heartbeat whilst populations of plaice, flounder and hermit crabs show 50% mortality after experiencing pressures in the range 120–150 ATM for 1 h.

Clearly deep sea organisms must have evolved microtubules, membranes and enzymes less sensitive to pressure than surface forms and presumably the sperm whale has the benefit of similar protection at the cellular level. How such baro-protection is achieved remains an intriguing question at present but it is certainly one which must be answered if man is even to start thinking of diving to the depths achieved by the whale.

7 Temperature Maintenance

A warm blooded animal experiences problems with regard to temperature maintenance as well as respiration during diving.

Potential difficulties arise because not only do some species experience wide temperature differences during annual migration between the tropics and high latitudes, but also in the differences that may be encountered during dives in tropical waters where the temperature can range between about 28°C at the surface to 4°C at 500 to 600 m (1640–1950 ft). Furthermore, water, owing to its greater thermal capacity and the effects of convection and conduction, is a more effective cooling agent than air. Conversely, the disposal of excess heat from the body by sweating is impracticable for an aquatic form since heat loss is achieved by the process of evaporation of sweat not by the secretion process. Marine species must, therefore, have provision for resolving the problems associated both with over-cooling and over-heating. Increased insulation is one answer to excessive heat loss and every layman knows that this is one function of the thick fatty 'blubber' found in marine mammals. The blubber can indeed be extensive, accounting for up to 40% of the body weight in small porpoises.

Measurements of temperature at different depths in the skin indicate the effectiveness of such thermal barriers. Thus, although the skin temperature of seals tends to be close to that of the ambient medium when the latter is in the temperature range 0–30°C, there is a steep temperature gradient in the sub-surface region so that for a seal in ice water the core body temperature is reached at a skin depth of about 5 cm.

The fins and flippers of cetaceans lack thick blubber layers and hence are potential sources of heat loss in cold waters. Such loss is, however, avoided by ingenious anatomical associations of the veins and arteries which tend to run parallel to one another so that it is possible for heat to be lost from the artery to the blood in the vein returning from the surface. By means of such counterflow, arterial blood is cooled before it reaches the periphery and the venous return from a fluke is warmed before passing to the body core (Fig. 7–1). That birds have a similar system is indicated by the low temperature of the legs from the start of the scaly region down to the feet.

Loss of heat from the surface is further limited by the increased peripheral resistance during a dive which restricts blood flow to the skin. It has been noted, for example, that the flippers of fur seals tend to be cool during a dive and warm after the animal surfaces. During a quiet dive in cool water seals may slowly lose heat and show a temperature drop.

However, the restriction of heat loss is sufficiently effective to be able to maintain heat balance without increase in activity and metabolic rate down to a temperature of 13°C (*Phoca vitulina*) or 5°C (gray seal). The still more arctic form, the harp seal, can even remain quiescent in ice water without the need to increase metabolic rate. In this respect seals have a considerable advantage over man, who suffers hypothermia quickly in cold water. A contributory feature to heat maintenance is of course the high blood metabolic rate of marine mammals already noted. If it were not for this high metabolic rate and the thermal barriers, a small porpoise would be expected to fall short of maintaining itself in heat balance by some six-fold if resting in water at 10°C, yet a porpoise can lie quietly in water at 7°C. Clearly the mechanisms are effective.

There are of course limits to the ability of some marine forms to balance heat loss without increasing muscular activity. Thus it is calculated that the Californian sea lion must swim to balance heat loss when at 0°C.

In warm waters it seems that the counter current systems are bypassed to allow access of warm blood to the body surfaces and so expedite loss of excess heat.

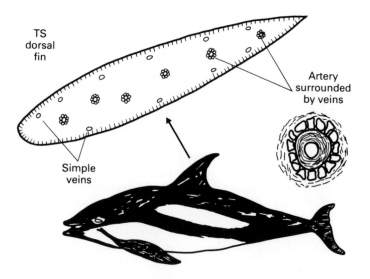

Fig. 7–1 Transverse section of the dorsal fin of the white-sided dolphin *Lagenorhynchus acutus* to show the juxtaposition of arteries and veins. (Freely adapted from SCHOLANDER and SCHEVILL, 1955.)

8 The Human Diver

Unlike the creatures discussed in the previous chapters, human beings have no natural need to enter the underwater world. Men go there either for advancement of their knowledge, exploitation of the available resources, military purposes, or simply for enjoyment, but only in comparatively recent times has it been possible to descend into the sea and stay there for more than a minute or two with a reasonable chance of returning to the surface in a healthy state. The reasons for needing the aid of modern technology become apparent when the nature of the problem is examined more closely.

8.1 Thermal exchange

Suppose for simplicity in the initial considerations that a man in swimming trunks is being lowered feet first from a fairly warm environment, 25°C, into a pool of fresh water at a temperature of 20°C. These are quite gentle conditions to contemplate but nevertheless two important points become immediately apparent. Firstly, due to its high thermal capacity, the water will feel cool and the body will take some minutes to adapt to the new environment before it begins to feel comfortable again; in fact a water temperature of 33°C is necessary to abolish shivering. Despite marked decreases in skin blood flow to reduce heat loss via the skin, and increases in metabolic rate to generate more heat, the body is unable to maintain itself in thermal balance if immersed in water at temperatures of 20°C, and indeed human survival is for many people reduced to a mere 15 min if they are immersed in sea-water at 0°C. Figure 8–1 shows approximate survival times for various water temperatures.

No great precision can be given to these data because people vary in their responses to cold water immersion, principally related to the amount of body insulation they possess in the form of subcutaneous fat. Thus fat people survive longer than thin people and women longer than men. As already noted, the ability of diving mammals to survive in cold waters is also closely related to the insulative value of their outer layer of fatty tissue, which is very much thicker than in the human (Chapter 7).

The measurement that can be quite precisely related to human survival is the deep body or 'core' temperature. Normally this is 37°C, but a reduction to 28°C causes loss of consciousness in all human beings. Examination of the surface temperatures of the oceans and lakes of the world reveals that most of them are considerably lower than 28°C and

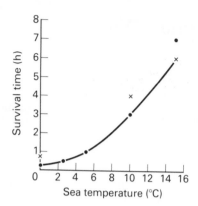

Fig. 8–1 Human survival time in various sea temperatures. The data are from two separate sources, one plotted ● and the other ×. A line has been drawn giving a reasonable average estimate of survival time for healthy adult (white) males.

therefore immersion can be a very serious hazard. Indeed it is now thought that drowning following loss of consciousness from hypothermia has been the greatest cause of death at sea.

The second gross observation which can be made when a body is lowered into water is that the water supports the weight of the body. Most normal men when passively lowered feet first into fresh water will float with just the top of their heads above the surface. However, a small proportion of men are negatively buoyant, and will continue to sink unless given added buoyancy. For all men, 'floaters' or 'sinkers', there is the same change in the hydrostatic pressure being exerted between the heart and the feet. In air it is necessary for the heart to pump with sufficient force to ensure that blood reaching the feet can be returned to the heart for recirculation. For a standing man there is a column of blood over a metre high to be supported and pumped round. When immersed in water this is no longer the case and the heart has considerably less work to perform to ensure adequate circulation in a fully immersed man. Thus there are complex changes in the cardiovascular system on immersion, some due to buoyancy effects, and some due to the response to changes in the rate of loss of heat via the skin.

8.2 Breathing underwater

In the early days the only known safe way to dive was to plunge into the water, holding one's breath, and by using swimming movements of the arms and legs it was possible to go to depths of the order of 30 m (100 ft) and return safely to the surface provided the oxygen present in the lungs on commencing the dive had not been reduced to a level which would cause loss of consciousness. This latter essential condition reduced the time underwater to a minute, or perhaps slightly more, in trained divers. The female Ama divers of Korea are the best known group of professional breath-hold divers in the world today, but underwater work is not normally practicable in this way.

Many attempts have been made to achieve greater and greater breath-hold dive depths and several have ended fatally, but it has been established that man can achieve depths near 100 m (330 ft) using this technique. On first consideration this would seem an impossible depth for a human being to achieve. The pressure of sea-water at 100 m is 11 atmospheres absolute. This means, by application of Boyle's Law, that the volume of gas present in the lungs when the diver left the surface has been reduced by a factor of eleven. His rib cage should therefore be crushed by the sea-water pressure on the chest, as it could not possibly sustain such a massive reduction in the volume of air in the lungs. In fact this does not happen because extra blood is brought into the pulmonary circulation and effectively increases the total volume of the lungs, thus helping to counteract the shrinkage in lung air volume caused by the increased sea-water pressure. As mentioned in earlier chapters, many diving mammals have a similar, more highly developed, form of adaptation to cope with the large changes involved in descending into the sea.

There is only one way whereby the volume of human lungs can be rendered independent of the depth of the dive. The pressure on the inside of the air passageways of the lungs, i.e. the lumen of the trachea, bronchi, bronchioles and alveoli, must be made the same, or very nearly the same, as the pressure on the outside of the chest wall. This requirement can readily be demonstrated by trying to breathe underneath the water through a rigid tube leading up to the surface. Once the length of tube connecting the mouth to the surface exceeds a few centimetres breathing becomes difficult or impossible. In order to avoid such pressure differentials it is necessary either to supply the lungs with a respirable gas under pressure, or to fill the lungs with some suitable liquid and, in effect, turn the lungs into gills. Clearly the first alternative appears the more acceptable and is the only technique used, at present, by the diver.

However, before dealing with the compressed gas solution to the problem of diving it is worth giving some attention to the more remote possibility of liquid breathing. An emulsion of fluorocarbon in thermostatted buffered saline solution can be used as a suitable liquid for mammals to breathe. The fluorocarbon, which is immiscible with water, has a high solubility for oxygen and the buffered saline in which it is suspended can effectively remove the carbon dioxide produced by the body tissues provided that the quantity of CO_2 does not exceed the amount that would be produced by light exercise. The reason for this limitation is that only about 5.5 l of liquid can be passed through the lungs every minute, due to the mechanical problem presented by attempting to breathe liquids instead of gases. A 'helium' diver, for example, breathes gas of density about 0.2 g l^{-1} at atmospheric pressure which is 5000 times less dense than suitable liquids. It is quite remarkable that mammalian lungs can ever function in such changed circumstances, and it is probable that some form of breathing assistance will have to be given to the human respiratory mechanism to keep it functioning for any length of time when breathings liquids.

The only way in use at present of avoiding the changes in lung gas volume that occur with changes in environmental pressure is to adjust the pressure of the gas being breathed by the diver. As a column of sea-water 10 m high exerts a pressure of 1 bar, then if the diver descends into the sea to a depth of 30 m he will need to be supplied with gas at a total pressure of 4 bar, i.e. 1 bar (approx.) at sea level plus 3 bar extra to counteract the sea-water pressure. The most readily available gas for him to breathe is, of course, air and therefore, intially, compressed air was used by all divers for underwater work.

The early pioneers developed two types of underwater apparatus. First there was the diving bell (Fig. 8–2) some of which could take several men down to the sea floor. It was necessary to make available a supply of fresh air, not only to keep the water from flooding the bell during descent, but also to keep the air fresh inside the bell when men worked in it.

Next came the 'helmet', 'hard hat', or 'standard dress' form of diving outfit. This consisted of a flexible waterproof suiting which held the arms, legs and torso. Attached to this suiting by a waterproof neck seal was a spherical copper helmet, fitted with a visor and air hose inlets and air outlet points, which held the diver's head and neck. Heavy boots were worn to ensure a safe, steady, standing position when working underwater. Vertical movement was generally accomplished by opening and closing the air pressure release valve, which in turn controlled the volume of air in the flexible suit, and hence the diver's buoyancy. Horizontal movement was achieved by walking or, more rarely, by pulling along with the hands. Clearly the development of the suit was a very formidable advance in underwater technique as it allowed the diver complete freedom of movement in his three-dimensional world.

It is now apparent why the aid of modern technology is necessary to ensure the safety of work underwater. The hoses connecting the diver to the surface must be able to withstand internal gas pressures at least equal to the pressure of sea-water where the diver is working, or they would collapse. Compressed gas must be pumped down the air hoses at a rate sufficient to ensure adequate ventilation of the helmet at all depths and this demands efficient, large air pumps. All these factors, and several more, require modern materials and techniques.

The history of diving apparatus, like the history of flying machines is quite fascinating and many devices which were clearly impractical or impossible were proposed and illustrated in old texts. Only the diving

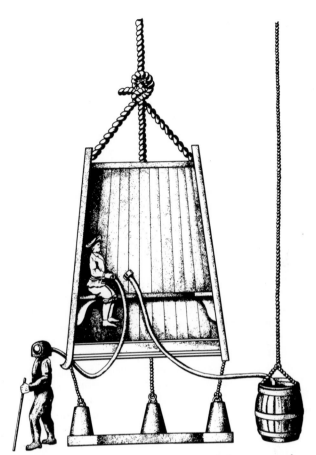

Fig. 8–2 Attempts had been made prior to 1700 to place men underwater for work purposes, but the first really practical system was the diving bell designed by Halley, of comet fame, in 1717. This was a truncated cone, of wooden construction, lead-lined and weighted to keep it vertical. A lens in the roof admitted light. Fresh air was supplied by lowering air-filled, lead-lined barrels each having a bung-hole in the top and bottom. Pressure of water was used to force air from the barrel into the bell by manipulating the leather tube loop.

bell, caisson, and the 'standard dress' evolved as the first practical propositions for underwater work. Nowadays there are complex variations of these basic systems, and mention will be made of these new approaches when discussing life support systems for divers.

As the diver descends into the sea, and the gas pressure supplied to him is increased to keep the breathing gas pressure equal to the sea pressure, this pressurized gas exerts three separate effects on the diver.

Firstly, there are volume changes in the body gas cavities other than the lungs. The inner ear is the most important of these, because if the air pressures on the outside and inside of the ear drum are not equal it may rupture. Fortunately, unless infection ensues, this is not generally a serious problem, as the ruptured drum will heal in a few weeks, and hearing is unimpaired. To avoid these painful distortions of the ear drum it is necessary to make sure that the Eustachian tube, which connects the inner ear with the pharynx, remains open. This is generally achieved by nipping the nostrils and creating a positive pressure in the upper airways of the pharynx and mouth which gives a sensation of 'popping' eardrums as the air is forced down the Eustachian tubes into the middle ear. If a diver cannot 'pop' or 'clear' his ears then he should not be allowed to dive. Inability to clear the ears is most often due to a cold or other infection of the upper respiratory tract.

Secondly, the compressed air increases in density and when the pressure exceeds about 6 bar (50 m, 165 ft, depth) breathing becomes too difficult to allow maximum physical exertion. This is a potentially dangerous situation and most codes of safe diving practice recommend that air diving should not be undertaken at depths exceeding 50 m. Increased air density also means increased body heat loss, altered voice characteristics, and numerous minor effects, e.g. inability to whistle. However, none of these latter changes give rise to concern. Indeed although compressed air is a better conductor of heat than air at atmospheric pressure it is nevertheless far less effective than sea-water at the same temperature. Consequently, divers often surround the body with a thin layer of air, trapped in their underclothing, which in turn is surrounded by the impervious flexible diving suit. This is termed the 'dry suit' method of diving and is by far the most comfortable diving suit for cold conditions.

Thirdly the compressed air dissolves in the blood as it flows through the lungs, and this changed blood is transported to the tissues. Divers are normally supplied with pure, very dry, air. Dryness prevents the dangers of ice formation due to the temperature drop in the pressure-reducing systems when supplying air to the diver. This dry air contains approximately 20% oxygen and 80% nitrogen and although these proportions alter slightly when the air enters the warm, water-saturated environment present in the lung alveoli, which also contain about 6% carbon dioxide, it is sufficiently accurate for the purposes of these preliminary considerations to say that the arterial blood flowing out of the lungs is in equilibrium with a partial pressure of about 0.2 bar oxygen and 0.8 bar nitrogen at atmospheric pressure. As the diver descends into the water the partial pressures of oxygen and nitrogen increase correspondingly, for example, at 5 bar total pressure (40 m, 130 ft, depth) the pressure of oxygen is 1 bar and of nitrogen 4 bar. However, because oxygen at a partial pressure of 0.2 bar is transported in a loose chemical combination with haemoglobin, the actual amount of extra oxygen transported at this greatly raised pressure is small (see Chapter 2), but the nitrogen which is inert, as far as blood is concerned, obeys Dalton's law of partial pressures, and therefore at 5 bar total pressure the arterial blood carries 5 times as much nitrogen as at 1 bar pressure. When this arterial blood reaches an active tissue the extra oxygen is quickly metabolized and tissue exchange may not be markedly altered, but if the extra mass of dissolved oxygen can actually supply most of the oxygen requirements of the tissue then there is little or no reduced haemoglobin available to aid carbon dioxide transport away from the tissues (see Chapter 2) and this can cause serious impairment of the normal tissue gas exchange processes. This will be referred to later, but does not represent a serious hazard to a diver during the course of his descent, due largely to the built-in delay factors of the body, i.e. time taken to circulate the blood to the tissues plus the time the tissues take to respond. This delay is normally about 5–7 min and if the diver descends at 30 m min^{-1}, which is a typical rate, he would be at an enormous depth before the problem became apparent.

8.3   Use of oxyhelium

Before the raised oxygen pressure affects the diver the increased partial pressure of nitrogen being supplied to the tissues will cause a major change in awareness. A short digression is necessary to explain why nitrogen causes this problem. If the fat (olive oil) solubilities of anaesthetic gases are plotted against their anaesthetic potency, it is apparent that an extremely good correlation exists (Table 8).

Table 8   The relationship between lipid solubility of gases and their narcotic potency.

Gas	Molecular weight	Lipid solubility (37°C) A	Relative Narcotic Potency B	A × B
			(Least narcotic)	
He	4	0.015	5.0*	0.075
Ne	20	0.019	3.6*	0.071
H$_2$	2	0.036	2.1*	0.076
N$_2$	28	0.067	1	0.067
A	40	0.14	0.43	0.060
Kr	84	0.43	0.14	0.060
Xe	131	1.70	0.04	0.068
			(Most narcotic)	

* It is not possible to separate with certainty the pressure itself and the narcotic effects hence the values given are reasonable estimates.

Although nitrogen has a relatively low fat solubility by comparison with chloroform, nitrous oxide, or even xenon, this can be enhanced to any desired level by raising the partial pressure of nitrogen. Thus the nitrogen concentration at normal atmospheric pressure can be regarded as a grossly sub-anaesthetic dose. When the pressure (concentration) of nitrogen is raised there seems to be no measureable effect on behaviour up to a pressure of about 4 bar. At that pressure the first signs of lack of concentration, over-confidence and irresponsibility begin to appear which are well known to the experienced air diver. These behavioural changes are often called 'nitrogen narcosis' or more popularly 'narks' or 'raptures of the deep'. There is no long silent period before the narcotic effects of nitrogen are noticed because the dissolved nitrogen is conveyed via the blood stream to the central nervous system and almost immediately saturates this well vascularized tissue with nitrogen at the new raised concentration. Unlike oxygen there is no metabolic delay because nitrogen does not play a part in the tissue chemistry. Thus there is only a circulatory delay of about 2 min before the full effects of raised nitrogen pressure are felt. In 2 min the average diver will have descended about 60 m (200 ft) into the sea, and at this pressure (7 bar) he is well beyond the 4 bar threshold at which the effects of nitrogen narcosis are first felt. Any further descent will place him in an increasingly hazardous situation. Thus air cannot be used deeper than about 60 m because thereafter most men will begin to behave irresponsibly.

Only if men can be compressed extremely rapidly is it possible to avoid the twin problems of narcosis and oxygen toxicity. Men have escaped from sunken submarines by rapidly flooding their escape chamber to depths as great as 180 m (600 ft) in 20 s, spent 3 to 5 s opening the escape hatch and getting out into the sea, and then with the aid of artificial buoyancy ascended through the sea-water back to the surface at a rate of about 2.5 m s^{-1}). Thus the whole escape procedure is completed in less than 2 min.

It is clear, then, that using compressed air the diver is limited to descents to 50 m depth, or at most 60 m, and unless some less dense, less narcotic, but nevertheless respirable gas mixture can be used, this would be the deepest safe diving depth. A non-narcotic gas must have a much lower fat solubility than nitrogen, and to give significant help to the breathing difficulties encountered at increased pressures it must be considerably less dense than air. Only helium and hydrogen have these desirable physical properties. However, as is well known, hydrogen is explosive when mixed with more than 4% oxygen, and it is therefore rarely used for deep diving. Several attempts have been made, and the physiological value of hydrogen as a deep diving gas is beyond dispute, but the explosive risks still act as an effective deterrent to its use.

The chemically inert, non-narcotic, and relatively cheap helium gas is now used for virtually all diving to depths greater than 50 m. Apart from its extensive use in nuclear physics, which has considerably reduced its cost, it is possible to obtain helium of a very high purity (99.995%), and there are no toxicological difficulties due to trace impurities even when breathing helium at great pressures. Helium was first used just prior to the Second World War, but it only became important as a diving gas during the period from 1965 onwards. At that time the exploitation of offshore resources, particularly oil, demanded prolonged underwater work in depths of water to the edge of the continental shelf, approximately 300 m (1000 ft).

When men first attempted descents breathing a gas mixture of oxygen and helium the most notable immediate changes, compared with previous experience on compressed air, were the dramatic loss of body warmth if the sea-water temperature was below 10°C and the remarkable voice distortion which was evident even at atmospheric pressure and which made the voice totally incomprehensible at depths greater than 60 m. The heat loss could be counteracted by wearing a heated diving suit and the voice could be rendered intelligible by using specially designed helium speech unscramblers.

However, once diving was taken to depths beyond 150 m (500 ft) a new effect began to emerge. Normally, as noted previously, divers descend to depth at 30 m min^{-1} and therefore it took 5 min to reach 150 m or 8 min to reach 240 m (800 ft). After 5 min compression to 150 m it was noticed that some men developed a trembling of the hands, which at first was thought to be due to nervousness or perhaps the inflow of helium into the lungs causing temporary retention of carbon dioxide. When compression at these rates was continued to 240 m every diver had the hand tremors, and some were even nauseated and disorientated. Clearly, this was not a psychological phenomenon and attempts were initiated to discover how pure, totally inert, helium gas could cause such obvious physical effects. In an early attempt to discover how deep men could descend on helium two volunteers reached 360 m (1200 ft) in a 2 h compression but were badly affected and had periods of micro-sleep. Their electroencephalograms showed significant depressions in the electrical activity of the brain and the experiments were terminated with the conclusion that whatever helium at pressure was doing, it was clear that men could not descend safely to depths in excess of about 350 m (1150 ft). All these changes caused by compression on helium were grouped under one heading and termed the High Pressure Nervous Syndrome (HPNS).

It was soon established that the onset of HPNS was very dependent upon the rate of compression. Thus if the divers took about 2 days instead of 2 h to compress to 360 m then the signs and symptoms of HPNS were almost absent. This was an important observation and demonstrated that, if the human body is given sufficient time during the course of the compression to adapt to the altered environment, apparently there are no ill-effects. On this basis, using specially selected volunteers, and with an extremely slow compression lasting 8 days, a depth of 610 m (2000 ft) has been safely reached. The difficulties of the compression phase have now been defined to depths as great as 600 m and it will next be considered how men can survive and work when brought to these various depths.

Why it is that a sperm whale can dive to 2000 m or more without apparently suffering from HPNS remains a mystery at present.

9 Man at Depth

The primary considerations on arrival at depth are the composition of the gases being breathed, the time on the bottom, and the depth of the dive. All these factors are interrelated and therefore the way in which the breathing gas composition influences the duration and depth of the dive will be examined. Air, as noted previously, cannot be safely used at depths in excess of 60 m (200 ft) because the density is too great for maximal exercise and furthermore the pressure of nitrogen causes behavioural changes. However, even at depths less than 60 m, air has a further limitation due to its oxygen content.

9.1 Oxygen toxicity

At the turn of the century it became established that prolonged breathing of oxygen at a pressure of one atmosphere was harmful to the lungs. It is now known that if the oxygen partial pressure exceeds 0.6 bar, prolonged breathing will lead to pleural effusion and lung oedema. Two intrepid experimenters once breathed pure oxygen at a pressure of about 1 bar for a period of 66 h and both became seriously ill and were lucky to survive.

If the partial pressure of oxygen is raised even further from 1 bar to 2 bar, the time to death for small animals decreases from 3–5 days to 19–24 h. Above 2 bar oxygen pressure the central nervous system begins to be affected, and convulsions supervene before the effects of the lung damage become apparent. For example, at 4 bar pressure most normal men could breathe pure oxygen for 30 min without ill-effects, but if asked to continue for 40 min, a large proportion would start involuntary muscular twitching, generally of the facial muscles, and expressively termed 'lips' by divers. This twitching tends to get more violent with the passage of time and spreads to other parts of the body, resulting in minor seizures. At this point the subject must be returned to air breathing, otherwise he will shortly lose consciousness and suffer violent convulsions. The generally agreed limits for oxygen breathing are given in Fig. 9–1.

A vast literature has accumulated but the aetiology of oxygen poisoning remains obscure. However, some important practical statements can be made. Breathing oxygen with carbon dioxide added causes an early onset of convulsions; similarly, heavy exercise or immersion in water or raising the metabolic rate also shorten the time to the onset of convulsions, whereas lowering the metabolic rate or using anaesthetic agents (and some tranquillizers) will delay the onset.

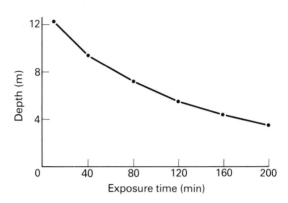

Fig. 9–1   Curve giving the normally accepted safe limits for breathing oxygen at pressure while exercising under water. (Based on data given in the *U.S. Navy Diving Manual*, 1975, U.S. Government Printing Office, Washington, D.C., and the *Royal Navy Diving Manual*, BR2806, with the permission of the Controller of H.M.S.O., London.)

It will now be realized that, for the air-breathing diver, the oxygen content of the air is adding a new set of constraints. For example at 40 m depth (130 ft) the partial pressure of oxygen in air is close to 1 bar, a concentration which, as we have seen, will have fatal results when breathed for several days, but will have measurable effects on lung function after only a few hours. The total duration of the dive, i.e. compression, time spent at depth, and decompression must therefore be assessed so that the permissible oxygen 'dosage' is not exceeded. In any estimations of safe oxygen usage it is also advisable to allow for a possible therapeutic recompression following the dive.

9.2   Saturation diving

The limitations of air or oxygen diving led to the use of mixtures of oxygen and helium for deep diving, but it became apparent that a 30 min dive at a depth of 140 m (450 ft) required about 10 h decompression to render it trouble-free for most divers. If the same dive were completed at say 150 m (500 ft) then 14 h decompression would be necessary. Clearly this type of diving could not be pursued as a practical proposition. The ratio of useful time on the bottom to the unprofitable time spent decompressing was shrinking too rapidly. Furthermore, only one dive a day was possible for any diver. Accordingly the technique of 'saturation' diving was introduced and nearly all diving work deeper than 60 m is now carried out using this technique, and it is indeed also used for a good deal of prolonged underwater work at depths as shallow as 30 m. Figure 9–2 shows a typical North Sea diving installation.

'Saturation' diving involves the diver living at a constant raised

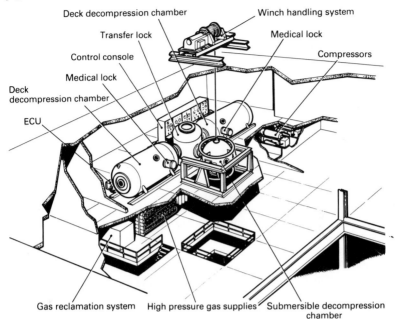

Deck decompression chamber   Winch handling system

Transfer lock   Medical lock

Control console

Medical lock   Compressors

Deck
decompression chamber

ECU

Gas reclamation system   High pressure gas supplies   Submersible decompression
                                                                                        chamber

Fig. 9–2   Schematic drawing showing the main features of a typical rig-based
saturation diving system.

pressure for a period of time sufficient to equilibrate all his tissues with
gas at the ambient pressure. This time is generally considered to be several
hours, but as yet no precise answer is possible. Once all his tissues have
equilibrated with the helium pressure then he has reached the maximum
decompression requirement, which cannot, in theory, be exceeded
however much longer he stays at depth. Put more quantitatively, if a diver
equilibrates all his tissues after a time t_1 at a pressure P, and his safe
decompression time is t_2, then if he stays a longer time, say αt_1 (where $\alpha > 1$)
the decompression time required is still t_2 and consequently the ratio of
useful time at depth to unusable time decompressing is

$$\frac{\alpha t_1}{t_2}.$$

Now as t_1 and t_2 are constant, for a given dive depth, this ratio can be
written $\alpha.k$, where k is t_1/t_2. Thus the ratio of useful time to useless time
can be made as big as one cares by increasing α.

The practical benefits of this technique are obvious but nevertheless
new problems are introduced. The requirement to stay for several days
under pressure necessitates supplying life support systems which will
work efficiently in an enclosed space at raised pressure. In essence it is the
problem of the manned space capsule compounded with the greatly

increased ambient pressures involved. The helium, for example, must be highly purified otherwise a concentration of say carbon monoxide of 1 part per 10^6 at 1 bar pressure, which is totally innocuous for prolonged breathing changes to an equivalent concentration of 30 parts per 10^6 when compressed to 30 bar (300 m, 1000 ft), and this is certainly not an innocuous level of carbon monoxide. Carbon dioxide is the principal undesirable contaminant gas to monitor and it is now accepted that a partial pressure of 0.005 bar (0.5% at 1 bar) should not be exceeded for very prolonged breathing. To measure reliably low levels of troublesome contaminants in an atmosphere at greatly raised pressures is a formidable technical problem.

A further requirement for the life support system is provision of adequate diver heating. At 1 bar pressure in calm air conditions the average lightly clothed man loses approximately 10% of his total body heat production via respiration, but at 180 m (600 ft) breathing oxyhelium the same man would lose as much as 50% via respiration. It must also be realized that the total heat loss, for a given ambient temperature, increases markedly by surrounding the body with helium at pressure. Therefore, the diver is not only losing more heat but the way in which his body loses this extra heat can change drastically with pressure. Most divers use hot water suits to overcome this extra heat loss, and also incorporate some form of heating for the inspired gas. Such hot water suits have the disadvantage that the diver can be scalded by defective or incorrectly used systems. However, they have a distinct advantage in offering a thermal capacity which delays the onset of hypothermia in emergencies when the hot water circulating system may fail. A reliable, practical, electrically heated suit has yet to be devised.

Living at pressure also entails breathing gases of abnormal densities for many days and it is not unreasonable to expect that the respiratory system may not cope indefinitely. In fact this does not seem to present a serious problem even as deep as 610 m (2000 ft) and experiments at 366 m (1200 ft) using neon (MW19) would lead one to suppose that respiratory problems will not be the limiting factor even as deep as 1500 m (4900 ft) using helium (MW4). The density of oxyhelium at 460 m (1500 ft) is roughly equal to that of air at 60 m (200 ft) which is the limit for safe air diving in open water, but if only light work is being demanded, it would be possible to go as deep as 100 m (330 ft) (see Fig. 9–3). This corresponds in density to helium gas at about 800 m (2600 ft). The reason why the work rate is not more seriously impaired with this extra increase in density is very complex and involves the following facts: (1) the proportions of laminar and turbulent flow alter, for a given gas flow rate, with increase in density; (2) the dynamic viscosity does not change with pressure; (3) the mass of gas to be moved increases with pressure; and (4) diffusivity of the physiologically important gases carbon dioxide and oxygen is affected by the alveolar gas environment.

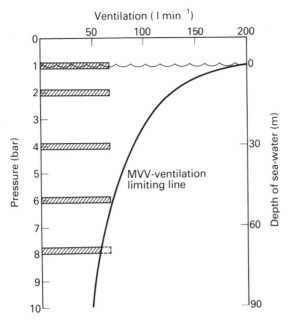

Fig. 9-3 Curve showing the relationship between maximum voluntary ventilation (MVV) and pressure of air. The horizontal shaded bars show the sustained maximum ventilation value for a healthy hard-working male. At a pressure of 6 bar (50 m gauge) a man is just able to work hard without reaching his maximum possible ventilation. At 8 bar he cannot perform hard sustained work, as he now requires more ventilation than his respiratory mechanisms can provide.

The designs of breathing apparatus vary from simple 'demand' valve systems on open circuit, as used by sports divers, to complex closed-circuit oxyhelium sets that maintain constant inspired oxygen partial pressures regardless of depth and work-rate.

9.3 Anaesthesia reversal

Unfortunately, although the respiratory system is remarkably adaptable to the changed environment of deep diving certain other body functions are not as accommodating. If the diver is taken to a depth greater than 300 m he begins to be affected by the pressure itself. Bouts of drowsiness, nausea, and sometimes even vomiting occur although the time taken to compress is sufficient to avoid the more obvious signs of HPNS. Also curiously disturbed are the subjective sensations of feeling warm or chilly, and divers tend to have poor quality sleep often with nightmares. The summation of all these physiological and psychological changes, which are now recognized as being due to effects on the peripheral vestibular mechanisms and central disturbances of cerebellar and brain stem function has halted the urge to go beyond 610 m (2000 ft) with human volunteers. Animals are therefore being used to plot the path ahead, but there is a formidable number of variables involved, such as body temperature, oxygen partial pressure, species of animal, time to reach pressure, time at pressure and action of pharmacological agents, particularly anaesthetics.

The use of liquid-breathing mammals has shown that all the major effects of HPNS are due to increasing the hydrostatic pressure and this has focused attention on the effects of pressure *per se*. It had been known for many years that applying pressure could restore the luminosity of luminous bacteria exposed to an anaesthetic agent and it was also similarly observed that if tadpoles were given a 2–5% ethanol/water medium in which to swim they quickly fell to the bottom of the vessel, but if a pressure of 150–200 bar was then applied the animals resumed swimming.

These simple pioneering observations were considerably extended later and it has now been established that mammals also show a reversal of anaesthetic effects with the application of pressure. The further very important additional observation was that whereas unanaesthetized mice were killed by application of a pressure of 120–150 bar, anaesthetized animals survived into a much higher pressure range of 160–240 bar. This pressure reversal of anaesthetic effect, while obviously having fundamental implications in the understanding of the action of anaesthetics, also holds out a hope of safely extending the depth to which human divers can attain.

From a practical standpoint it does seem that for man to reach pressures as great as 80 bar (800 m) many days, possibly weeks, will be required. Failure to withstand these large pressures generally manifests itself, in animals, by the onset of convulsions. Clearly this means that man must proceed cautiously to greater depths if he is to avoid damage to his body.

10 Returning to the Surface

Robert Boyle in 1670 observed a bubble in the eye of a viper subjected to a much reduced air pressure in his 'pneumatic machine'. This was the first demonstration of the dangers attendant upon too great a drop in ambient pressure. Many years later, when diving, tunnel and caisson work became possible, it was realized that these workers were acquiring dissolved gas in their tissues which could, following too rapid a return to atmospheric pressure, cause the formation of free gas, as with Boyle's viper. Analysis of the free gas present in the blood and tissues showed that it consisted of approximately 95% nitrogen. The oxygen content of the air was having little or no effect because, as mentioned earlier, oxygen is metabolized by tissues and it is therefore very difficult to sustain excess tissue concentrations of oxygen for very long. Obviously pure oxygen would be the gas of choice for diving if it were not for the unfortunate fact of oxygen poisoning.

10.1 Decompression sickness

The return to atmospheric (surface) pressure after a dive must be conducted in such a way that, if any gas is released, its quantity should be small enough not to cause trouble. If too much gas is released, decompression sickness ensues and this can take any one (or more) of several forms. The mildest form is skin itching or mottling; the severest form is when large numbers of bubbles in the blood cause blockage of the pulmonary and cardiac circulation, expressively termed 'chokes' by the diver, which is a rapidly fatal condition. In between these two extreme forms of acute decompression sickness are the more commonly encountered manifestations such as pains felt in joints' or sometimes deeply in muscles termed 'bends', paralysis of one or more limbs, and various other less common manifestations such as vertigo, deafness, visual phenomena and paraesthesiae. In all cases of decompression sickness the remedy is prompt recompression. This never fails, and a typical recommended recompression procedure for air divers is given in Table 9. Only if recompression is delayed will the therapy be liable to fail, the simple explanation being that the released bubbles have caused such tissue damage that recompressing them to an asymptomatic size is unable to repair the tissue.

In order to avoid acute decompression sickness it is necessary to observe the conditions which cause and cure the problem. A summary of these conditions follows Table 9.

Table 9   Air recompression therapy table for treating serious*
cases of decompression sickness.

Gauge depth (m)	Stoppages (h and min)	Elapsed time (h and min)	Rate of ascent
50	2 h	0000–0200	5 min between stop-
42	30 min	0205–0235	pages throughout
36	30 min	0240–0310	
30	30 min	0315–0345	
24	30 min	0350–0420	
18	6 h	0425–1025	
15	6 h	1030–1630	
12	6 h	1635–2235	
9	12 h	2240–3440	
6	4 h	3445–3845	
3	4 h	3850–4250	
Surface		4255	

* Serious means involvement of the brain, spinal cord, or
cardiovascular system leading to signs and symptoms such as
unconsciousness, inability to move arms or legs, loss of speech or
hearing, visual disturbances, hypersensitivity or anaesthesia of
skin, difficulty of breathing, choking sensations. When using
recompression procedures such as those given above the main
sources of failure arise from divers not reporting symptoms, or
from delays in treatment because divers wait to see whether the
troubles will go away.

(a) All mild 'bends' cases will resolve if treated promptly by
recompression.

(b) Short duration dives can safely be carried out at greater depths than
long duration ones. This suggests that a quantity of gas is involved. In
fact it is found that if P is the pressure of the dive and t its duration,
then the equation $P_\sqrt{} t = K$ (where K is constant) quite adequately
describes the known data on air provided t does not exceed 100 min.
When P is measured in feet of sea-water K is 500. So, for example, if
P = 100 then t = 25, i.e. if a diver descends quickly to a depth of 100 ft
under the sea, and remains at that depth for 25 min, it is safe to return
back quickly to surface (atmospheric) pressure. If the diver stayed
longer than 25 min he would exceed the K value of 500 and there
would be a definite risk of decompression sickness should he return
quickly to the surface. Similarly if the depth were 50 ft then as
$50\sqrt{t} = 500$ the just safe (threshold) value of t would be 100 min. Using
metric units K is 150.

(c) Following prolonged exposure to pressure it is observed that the threshold (just safe) pressure for rapid return to atmospheric pressure is greater when breathing helium-oxygen, than nitrogen-oxygen (air) and this is greater again than argon-oxygen. It is the inert gas content of the breathing mixture which is responsible for provoking attacks of decompression sickness and it is therefore some physical property of these inert gases which decides the order of sensitivity.

(d) In most cases of mild bends there is a trouble-free waiting period prior to the onset of bends. This waiting period can vary from a few minutes to several hours.

(e) Some forms of diving can lead to adaptation or acclimatization which increases the resistance of the divers to attacks of mild decompression sickness.

(f) There is an asymmetry between the uptake and elimination of inert gases by the body during normal compression and decompression procedures. Gas enters more rapidly during compression than it leaves during decompression.

(g) Prolonged exposures to pressure followed by rapid decompression to a new just safe level are feasible up to great pressures, at least 500 m (1640 ft). The relationship between the pressure of exposure (P_1) and the pressure to which it is safe to decompress (P_2) is of the form $P_1 = aP_2 + b$, where a and b are constants for a particular breathing gas composition and a particular form of decompression sickness. For example to avoid limb pains (bends) when breathing compressed air a is 1.36 and b is 3.4 when using the metre of sea water as the pressure unit. At 10 m of sea-water pressure (P_1), which is exactly 1 bar, then the subatmospheric pressure to which it is just safe to ascend (P_2) is 4.8 m of sea-water or 0.48 bar.

(h) Oxygen breathing at pressure will 'wash out' inert gases dissolved in the tissues, and this considerably helps the speed of decompression. However, oxygen at pressure can be toxic, and therefore it can only be fully exploited in the lower pressure range (20 m, 66 ft, or shallower). The permitted oxygen 'dosage' must not be exceeded, as was mentioned when discussing air diving limitations. Sometimes when a diver has been breathing oxyhelium at pressure it is possible to change him to another breathing mixture, e.g. air, and this has been shown to have temporary advantages in the speed of decompression. The reason given is that helium, being a small mobile molecule, moves out of the relevant tissues more rapidly than the larger more slowly diffusing molecule nitrogen moves in, hence for a while there is a drop in total inert gas present and this means the ambient pressure can be lowered more rapidly without causing decompression sickness. Once again this technique can present difficulties. If the diver breathes the air through a mask for a long period with his body surrounded by oxyhelium, the skin and other exposed surfaces have a full concentration of dissolved helium, and the local blood supply brings up a full quota of dissolved nitrogen from his breathing gas. This can cause an excess of total dissolved gas in these tissues and give skin rashes, due to bubble formation, even at a constant ambient pressure.

(j) Osteonecrosis (bone necrosis, aseptic necrosis of bone) can occur as a result of hyperbaric exposures. This condition is only detectable radiologically many months after the causative exposure. In a small number of cases those bone lesions which are near the moving surfaces of joints can develop and create serious mechanical weakness leading to a painful collapse of the joint surface. It does now seem that osteonecrosis is related to the adequacy of decompression, although men without any history of overt attacks of bends can nevertheless show osteonecrotic lesions and conversely men who have had numerous attacks of the bends are sometimes quite free from any such bone disorders.

10.2   Bubble formation

From these basic agreed facts it is necessary to create a quantitative approach to solve the practical problem of deciding the pressure/time course that a diver should follow during his decompression in order to avoid decompression sickness and yet be economical of time. This problem has not been satisfactorily solved because the main bases for calculation are not yet known. The only point of common agreement is that a bubble, or separated gas, is the primary cause of most forms of acute decompression sickness, including the bends. Left for speculation are the following further points.

(a) Is a gas nucleus always present physiologically, either in 'crevices' in tissue walls or perhaps from vortical motion of the blood in the heart? If so, no decompression can be undertaken following a dive without the presence of a gas phase in the tissues or circulation.

(b) Is there a small permissible pressure drop that will not cause bubble formation? It could be supposed that as there must be an oxygen partial pressure in the breathing mixture to sustain life then a rapid drop nearly equal to this oxygen pressure could be sustained without causing the inert gas to come out of solution. Oxygen, as noted previously, is metabolized away and therefore creates a partial unsaturation of the gases in the tissues.

(c) Is there a permitted excess total dissolved gas pressure which the tissues can sustain before bubble formation? Anything less than this critical permitted excess pressure has a vanishingly small risk of causing decompression sickness, whereas any greater excess pressure has a near certainty of causing decompression sickness. Most decompression procedures in use today invoke this latter concept.

Even if answers to these three questions regarding the origin of the bubble were known, there is still no agreed view on where the bubble is to be found. Various ideas are advanced.

(i) The relevant bubbles are intravascular and are first formed either in the arterial circulation or, perhaps, in the venous.
(ii) The relevant bubbles are extravascular and are formed in interstitial fluid or intracellularly.
(iii) The relevant bubbles are peripheral, or central with stimuli giving referred pain.

Once again, even if both the source and site were settled it is not really known how inert gas molecules dispose themselves in the relevant tissues. Two major views are held, one supposing that the rate of elimination of excess dissolved gas molecules is largely dependent upon their rate of diffusion through tissue spaces, the other concept being that elimination is largely a function of the blood flow through the tissue. Many of the disagreements given above are upon matters of basic physiological knowledge and would prevent underwater work if answers had to be obtained before sensible decompression procedures could be suggested, but using processes of trial and error optimum diving schedules are slowly being evolved.

Some of the questions posed above have received considerable attention, and it is to be hoped that firm answers are not too far away. For example, ultrasound techniques have been used to demonstrate the presence of gas bubbles in the diver's circulation during decompression. While, therefore, it can be stated that often there are bubbles post-dive, it is not yet known how relevant these bubbles are to the decompression problems, because even when they are shown to be present in large numbers, it does not always mean that the diver is about to have an attack of decompression sickness; mostly they remain asymptomatic. To observe the formation, growth and decay of the relevant bubble, or bubbles is going to be a formidable task.

10.3   Post-decompression

Since 1888 it has been suspected that there is a connection between working in compressed air and certain forms of bone damage which appear many months or even years after cessation of work. Perhaps the most interesting of the early accounts was the finding of osteonecrosis in three survivors who escaped from a submarine (HMS *Poseidon*) which had sunk in 1936 in 36 m (120 ft) of water off the coast of China. Their bone lesions resulted from only one exposure to high pressure air of approximately three hours duration inside the flooded compartment of the sunken submarine, followed by rapid ascent to the surface during escape. All the survivors suffered badly from decompression sickness on surfacing, but they all recovered from their acute problems only to be stricken twelve years later by the chronic bone disorder. Indeed, prior to 1947, it was thought that such an attack of acute decompression sickness (bends, or paralysis, etc.) was a necessary precursor for the appearance of these chronic bone lesions. However, large radiographic surveys have revealed the significant, and rather disturbing, fact that osteonecrosis can occur in a significant percentage of men who have no history of being treated for decompression sickness. A typical analysis is given in Table 10.

Table 10   Comparison of the incidence of bends and bone lesions in human divers.

	Bends	No bends	Total
Men with bone lesions	17	21	38
Men without bone lesions	25	160	185
TOTAL	42	181	223

It is generally believed that the cause of diver's and compressed air workers' osteonecrosis is nitrogen or helium bubbles released as a result of inadequate decompression, producing blockage of nutrient vessels in the bone which leads to absorption of bone, perhaps collapse, and later to some extent, new bone formation.

Such chronic after-effects of exposure to pressure led to enquiries into how soon it is possible to detect post-dive changes.

Work has been instituted to follow behavioural, haematological and biochemical changes occurring during the exposure to pressure to see if any of these changes persist in the post-exposure period, as well as ascertaining whether the post-dive period has changes other than the radiologically detectable osteonecrosis.

It is now clear that all the behavioural changes seen under high pressures of nitrogen or helium are entirely reversible with pressure and disappear during the decompression phase. However, there are some changes which occur and their effects are still measurable several days after the dive has terminated. In 1972 it was shown that although, not altogether surprisingly, there were measurable changes in a variety of blood constituents immediately following a dive there were some effects, in particular the platelet count, which diminished to a minimum value two or three days after the dive and took between a week and ten days before returning to pre-dive levels. This was the first demonstration that an apparently quite safe, trouble-free, air dive of only one hour's duration at 30 m (100 ft) depth could cause after-effects which persisted for several days (Fig. 10–1).

The implications of these findings are not yet properly understood. The practical facts are that men can repeatedly perform exposures to compressed air for hundreds of times over periods of several years and the only long term risk uncovered so far is that of osteonecrosis, which,

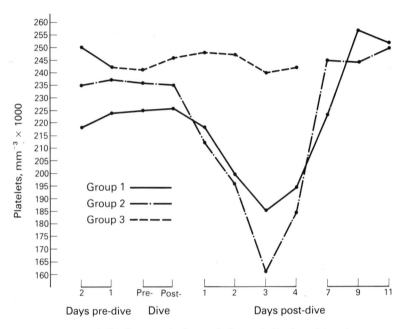

Fig. 10–1 Typical platelet count before and after a 1 h dive breathing air at 30 m. Groups 1 and 2 are diving groups and are compared with a non-diving control group (Group 3). The dramatic fall in the count between 2 and 4 days post-dive is clearly seen.

fortunately, generally remains asymptomatic and leaves the man functionally normal. Whether oxyhelium diving causes any similar chronic after-effects is not yet known as there are no divers who have dived using only pure oxyhelium gases throughout their working life. All divers tend to learn their diving expertise using conventional air-breathing techniques before transferring to the more complex requirements of synthetic gas mixture breathing. Furthermore many decompression schedules employ air breathing during the lower pressure stages, from about 35 m (116 ft) to the surface. Thus no divers can claim to be free from the possibility that post-dive effects are due to breathing compressed air.

It does seem that, after several years' experience with deep oxyhelium diving (150 m, 500 ft or deeper), there are no new chronic problems emerging, and indeed it would seem that this new era of deep diving is less troublesome in this respect than that which ushered in the era of compressed air diving, caisson and tunnel working.

10.4   The future

Already man can survive underwater for indefinite periods at depths as great as 500 m (1640 ft) and in this respect has far surpassed the ability of all other mammals, but the price paid in time, descending and ascending safely, is very considerable and such diving is becoming increasingly more difficult to accept as a practical proposition. Nevertheless, there is little doubt that if a man can be brought in person to the scene of action, this is preferable in the current state of technology. Underwater, remote-controlled devices stand in the same kind of relationship to man, as man does to the dolphin. Machines are superior in certain respects, such as depth capability but lack the manoeuvrability and versatility of men. By investing much more effort it is possible that both men and machines can satisfactorily overcome their respective major weaknesses. In the meantime, many thousands of human beings liberated by modern technology that gave them the 'demand' valve, high pressure gas cylinders, flexible neoprene suits, etc., will continue to enjoy returning to the environment from which life on earth began.

11 Summary

The ability of specialist diving forms to remain for extended periods below the surface can be attributed to a number of factors among which are: (1) enlarged intial oxygen carriage in the body due to the high O_2 capacity of the blood and extended blood volume; (2) vasoconstriction of the blood vessels leading to 'non-essential' tissues which thus conserves oxygen for aerobic tissues; (3) the ability to build up a large oxygen debt through accumulation of lactic and other organic acids in the muscles; (4) the development of some ability (extensive in reptiles) of the brain and heart to tolerate reduced oxygen levels and derive energy from anaerobic processes; (5) evolution of mechanisms providing for both facultative and involuntary bradycardia to an extended degree; (6) insensitivity of the respiratory centres to CO_2.

Morphological modifications contributing to the survival of animals undertaking deep dives are the collapsible lungs, presence of extensive rete mirabile in the thorax and sinuses which can be filled with blood to act as pressure-matching devices, and the provision of pressure-protected arterial and venous supplies to the head.

Many of the problems experienced by man when diving are associated with the fact that he is supplied with gas pressurized to a level equivalent to the hydrostatic pressure at the working level. When breathing air, he will experience problems of nitrogen narcosis and respiratory embarrassment at depths greater than about 55 m (180 ft), and nitrogen bubbles forming in the blood and tissues may cause 'bends' if surfacing occurs too quickly. Pure oxygen should not be used in extended dives to depths greater than about 8 m (26 ft) because of the risk of onset of acute or chronic oxygen toxicity. Substitution of helium-oxygen mixtures can be used to overcome nitrogen narcosis and respiratory difficulties and human simulated dives on appropriate mixtures have been successfully accomplished to 610 m. A slow rate of increase in pressure is necessary for dives over about 250 m (820 ft) if the severity of the High Pressure Nervous Syndrome (HPNS) is to be reduced. Some success has been achieved in experiments with animals by the use of narcotic gases to counter HPNS.

Further Reading

ANDERSEN, H. T. (1966). Physiological adaptations in diving vertebrates. *Physiol. Rev.*, **46**, 212–43.

ANDERSEN, H. T. (Ed.) (1969). *The Biology of Marine Mammals*. Academic Press, New York.

ANGELL JAMES, J. and de BURGH DALY, M. (1972). In: *The Effects of Pressure on Organisms* edited by M. A. Sleigh and A. C. MacDonald. *Symp. Soc. exp. Biol.*, **26**. Cambridge Univerity Press, Cambridge.

BENNETT, P. B. and ELLIOTT, D. H. (Ed.) (1975). *The Physiology and Medicine of Diving*. Baillière Tindall, London.

CLARKE, M. R. (1978). Buoyancy control as a function of the spermaceti organ in the sperm whale. *J. mar. biol. Assoc. U.K.*, **58**, 27–71.

DUGAN, J. (1965). *Man under the Sea*. Macmillan, New York.

KOOYMAN, G. L. (1972). Deep diving behaviour and effects of pressure in reptiles, birds and mammals. In: *The Effects of Pressure on Organisms*, edited by M. A. Sleigh and A. C. MacDonald. *Symp. Soc. exp. Biol.*, **26**, 295–311. Cambridge University Press, Cambridge.

MILES, S. (1962). *Underwater Medicine*. Staples Press, London.

NORRIS, K. S. (ed.) (1966). *Whales, Dolphins and Porpoises*. University of California Press, Berkeley and Los Angeles.

SCHLIEPER, E. J. (1962). *Whales*. Hutchinson, London.

SCHOLANDER, P. F. (1962). *Harvey Lectures*, **57**, 92–110. Academic Press, New York.

SCHOLANDER, P. F. (1965). Animals in aquatic environments: diving mammals and birds. In: *Adaptation to the Environment*. pp. 729–40. Section 4 of *Handbook of Physiology*, edited by D. B. Dill, E. F. Adolf and C. G. Wilber. American Physiological Society, Washington, D.C.